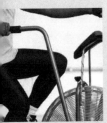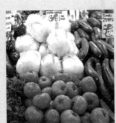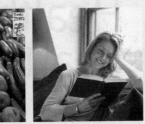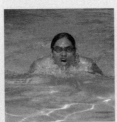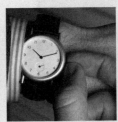

brilliantideas

one good idea can change your life...

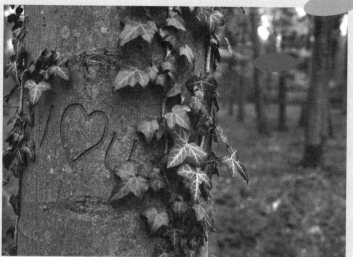

Healthy
heart

Keep your ticker happy

Dr Ruth Chambers

CAREFUL NOW...

All the ideas here are intended to inform, entertain and provoke your thinking. They're for general information only, and should not be treated as a substitute for medical advice from your own doctor or other healthcare professional. While every effort has been made to provide accurate and up-to-date information, medical science is constantly evolving. Neither the author nor the publisher can be held responsible or liable for any loss or claim arising out of the use, or misuse, of the suggestions made in this book; we don't know your specific circumstances and so we're not suggesting any specific course of action for you to follow. It makes sense for you to weigh up the choices available carefully and to decide what action, if any, you might take; after all, it's your health and it's your life. If in doubt, you should always consult your doctor for individualised health and medical advice.

Although the contents of this book were checked at the time of going to press, the world keeps moving as does the world wide web. This means we can't guarantee the contents of any of the websites mentioned in the text.

Copyright © The Infinite Ideas Company Limited, 2005

The right of Ruth Chambers to be identified as the author of this book has been asserted in accordance with the Copyright, Designs and Patents Act 1988.

First published in 2005 by
The Infinite Ideas Company Limited
36 St Giles
Oxford
OX1 3LD
United Kingdom
www.infideas.com

A CIP catalogue record for this book is available from the British Library.

ISBN 1-904902-57-X

Brand and product names are trademarks or registered trademarks of their respective owners.

Designed and typeset by Baseline Arts Ltd, Oxford
Printed by TJ International, Cornwall

Brilliant ideas

Brilliant features

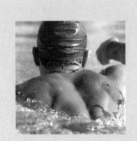

Each chapter of this book is designed to provide you with an inspirational idea that you can read quickly and put into practice straight away.

Throughout you'll find four features that will help you get right to the heart of the idea:

- *Here's an idea for you* Take it on board and give it a go – right here, right now. Get an idea of how well you're doing so far.

- *Try another idea* If this idea looks like a life-changer then there's no time to lose. *Try another idea* will point you straight to a related tip to enhance and expand on the first.

- *Defining idea* Words of wisdom from masters and mistresses of the art, plus some interesting hangers-on.

- *How did it go?* If at first you do succeed, try to hide your amazement. If, on the other hand, you don't, then this is where you'll find a Q and A that highlights common problems and how to get over them.

Introduction

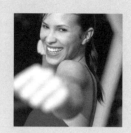

Unsure about how to keep your heart healthy? Then these 52 ideas are just the medicine for you. They're easy and fun to read, and you'll want to try the ideas here because they're presented in an engaging and entertaining way. I know you've had enough of being hectored and told what to do; that sort of tack doesn't work anyway. You'll only get yourself into a healthy way of life if you want it enough.

You can take the ideas out of sequence; they don't run from front to back. After all, you can do a good number of them in parallel, all at once. But don't risk missing chunks out; otherwise, just imagine, the three or four vital tips that could literally save your life, or at least mean that you stay healthy for longer, could be the very parts you pass over.

Reading these brilliant ideas, you'll be stunned by the number of things you can do, all by yourself, to help your heart. It's not rocket science. Much of the stuff you'll know already. But you won't have put it into practice consistently – yet. It's never too late, either. You'll see from the ideas on stopping smoking just how quickly your body can right itself after years of abuse. Get every one of your bad little habits exposed, so that you can track and blitz yours – now and forever.

So let's see how you'll go forwards. Some information here you'll read so often you'll know the text by heart (sorry!). You'll put your heart into devising and sticking with an exercise regime. If you relapse in your fitness plan, your heart will sink but you won't lose heart – you'll promise to get back on track from the bottom of your heart. You'll aim for the body weight your heart desires. You may have a heart-to-heart with your personal trainer, then set yourself a realistic goal. When you're nearing your target and getting on those scales, your heart will be in your mouth. And after your change of heart, you won't recognise yourself: you'll be eating sensibly, exercising frantically, stamping out smoking and limiting alcohol drastically.

This book is for you if you've got a healthy heart – as far as you know – in order to keep it that way. It's for you, too, if you have problems with your heart. (Physical ones, that is. If you've romantic problems, then hold this book in an obvious way in a public place and you'll probably get a queue of people coming up to chat to you just to get a chance of looking more closely at it – you may even meet your perfect partner by using this approach.) You can take the same type of measures to keep your heart healthy as you do to restore or maintain its health; it's just that you might have more capacity to go further if you're not troubled by ill health. But if you've had any sort of health scare, even one that turned out to be unfounded, you'll probably be well motivated to follow the information and advice here and apply it to yourself.

Let's look at things from your heart's perspective. You can't treat it in isolation; only a pathologist doing a post-mortem can do that. Your heart is inextricably linked to your bloodstream (as you can see, my medical training has paid off with detailed knowledge like this) and that means that you have to pay attention to keeping your blood pressure down to normal levels to optimise conditions for your heart to thrive. Your bloodstream passes round your body picking up all sorts – fur and debris. You don't want any of that so, as vacuuming your blood vessels is not an option, you'll have to stick to a low-fat diet or take statin drugs to clean up for you. Your heart lives in parallel with your lungs – and when there's a pressure build up there, your heart suffers too. Drugs that might help your heart, like aspirin, can cause troubles elsewhere, troubles like bringing on a stomach ulcer that bleeds into your gut... I'll look at all of these in the 52 ideas.

So, your heart is sitting there in your body all unsuspecting. It doesn't know what you've got in store for it. It hasn't yet experienced the regular exercise. It's still struggling with over-rich blood cascading through it. It's still knocked out by an overdose of alcohol when you binge too often (and once is too often, I'm afraid). It is still huffing with too little oxygen as carbon poisons trail through it. It'll seem as though your heart is reborn when you turn these 52 brilliant ideas into reality.

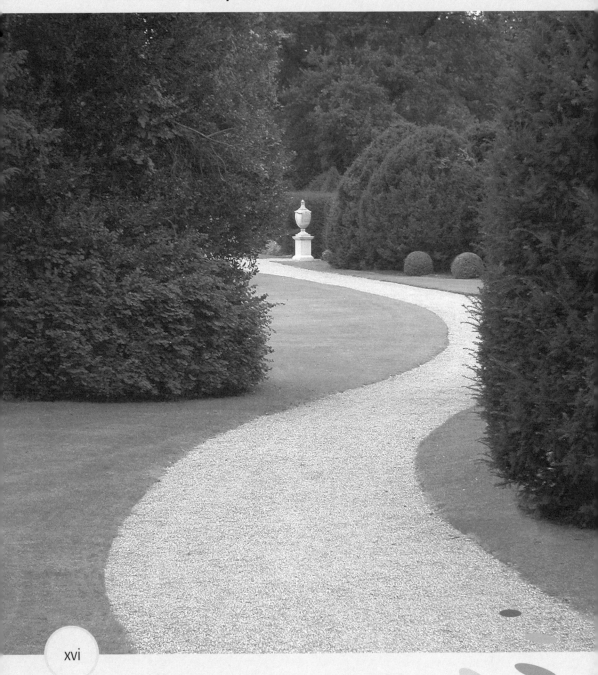

Appearances aren't always deceptive

What do you do when you've got lines round your mouth and eyes and your face looks like it belongs to a grandparent?

Your physical appearance shows what's going on inside your body and mind. So it's not just shallow to worry about it – and investing in your health will benefit your appearance...

The more you hit society's top ratings for attractiveness, the more people will want your company, and people with close and loving relationships have fewer heart problems, physically as well as romantically. So being your ideal weight and glowing with health should boost your personal relationships – and directly benefit the condition of your heart.

Have a direct debit for your gym membership, and go! Someone with well-toned muscles is attractive, whatever their age, compared to someone with flabby arms or thighs. And with regular exercise and a healthy balanced diet, you'll look radiant and bursting with vitality: unless, that is, it's straight after a heavy workout in the gym when, fair enough, you might be a bit of a sweaty mess. So don't risk squandering all your spare cash on going out clubbing, buying new clothes and beauty products; prioritise what you spend on your health and fitness.

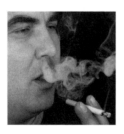

SPOT THE SMOKER

Well, if you do look like one of your grandparents, then you could always be the new face of the stop-smoking lobby. Quite apart from all the purely health-related problems it brings, smoking also narrows the blood vessels nourishing your skin. So as these blood vessels become thinner and more fragile, you end up with broken thread veins. Years of pursing your lips as you draw on cigarettes lead to furrows and lines around your mouth and eyes, more pronounced because smoke damages the elastic tissue of your skin. This is why smokers are often prematurely wrinkled. In addition, the yellow discoloration of your fingers, teeth and nails are the giveaway that you're a smoker. OK, smoking does curb your appetite and helps you keep your weight down. But there are other ways of doing that – like not eating as much and exercising more...

DON'T BANK ON FATTY DEPOSITS

Get your cholesterol levels down and hopefully you'll avoid those telltale fatty deposits near your eyes. But it's not just that – the heavier you are, the more likely you'll be to have heart problems as well as other diseases, all because of your excess weight. It's the size of your waist or your waist to hip ratio that can predict whether you'll have heart problems. So before you let your belt out another notch, get out the tape measure. If you're a man with a waist of at least 94 cm (37 in) or, even worse, of more than 102 cm (40 in), your health's at risk. Similarly, if you're a woman with a waist measurement of at least 80 cm (32 in) or, worse, more than 88 cm (35 in), then your health's at risk too. You've more chance of high blood pressure, having a heart attack or angina, or a high cholesterol level, all depending on how fat you are.

Now you know about the dangers of being fat, especially round the middle of your trunk, look at IDEA 11, *Battle of the bulge*, for more clues on how to lose weight and keep it off.

Try another idea...

RIGHT TO BE WRONG

There may be a price to pay for taking drugs to enhance your attractiveness. If you're taking hormone replacement therapy in an attempt to keep yourself looking younger, rather than for other reasons, then you should know that a few women will end up having a heart attack or a stroke that they wouldn't have had otherwise. If you're taking steroids illegally to boost your chances in athletics or sport, you could be triggering high blood pressure or diabetes, both of which could affect your heart. And taking Viagra to impress your partner or disguise your erection problems can make any heart problems worse.

'For the Lord seeth not as man seeth: for man looketh on the outward appearance, but the Lord looketh on the heart.'
The Bible

Defining idea...

Q **My bloke does look pretty red in the face. It seems to be his
natural look. Do you think he might have a problem with his heart?**

A *Some people's colour is naturally high. But could he be drinking too much
alcohol? That could give him a red complexion, especially after a binge
when the alcohol has dilated his blood vessels so there's more blood near
the surface of his skin. People who are unfit can look red in the face after
unaccustomed exercise – you could treat him to membership of a gym
where he'd have a personal assessment before starting anything.*

Q **How does stress and anxiety affect people's appearance? Does
your face mirror your feelings?**

A *Yes, you'll get worry lines on your face and that's not all. Your stress will
have an effect on your heart and general health. As well as that, the knock-
on effects may be eating more and smoking for comfort – and that'll affect
your appearance too. Women's faces might seem to age quicker, but women
have the last laugh as men's hearts age more quickly than women's – they
lose heart-pumping power at a younger age.*

Q **How can cosmetic surgery can help my appearance?**

A *Cosmetic treatment could backfire if your heart's not strong enough to
withstand the anaesthetic or surgery. Find out the risks first before you
agree to anything. Stick with mainstream health care and don't be tempted
by lower price deals in back-street clinics. Misplaced injections and excessive
doses of Botox can paralyse distant muscle groups – including your heart
muscles, giving you a heart attack or irregular heart rhythm.*

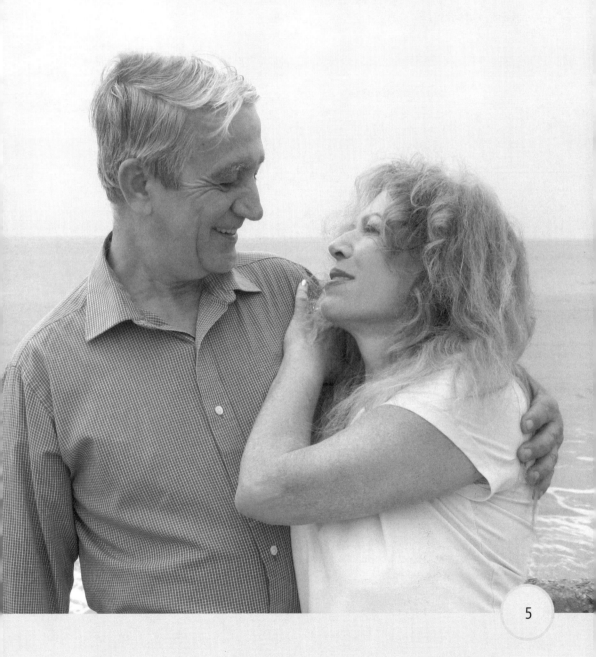

2

Cutting your risks

Help yourself! What, to another ciggie, or just one more chocolate or whisky? No – really help yourself by stopping smoking, eating a healthy diet, exercising regularly and avoiding too much alcohol.

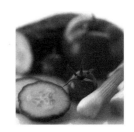

Risk is a chance of things going wrong. Cutting your risks is about making it less likely you'll have heart problems, or ensuring that they'll be more minor if you do.

DO YOU REALISE...

Some of your risks of having heart disease or complications, you can change: like having high blood pressure or smoking cigarettes. Others you can't: like being male, or who your parents are. Some risks, like diabetes, you can reduce with a healthy lifestyle. Some, like blood clots, you might minimise by taking aspirin every day. Think of the risks of being overweight or obese. Women who are obese are twelve times more likely to develop diabetes, four times more likely to suffer from raised blood pressure and three times more likely to have a heart attack. Obesity is risky for men too, though not quite as much.

Draw up a risk assessment for yourself now – gauging all the sources of stress and risks to your heart in your life. Include how stressful or high profile your job is, how often you eat out or buy fat-laden takeaways: all your bad lifestyle habits. Have you got a mistress or a toy boy in tow burdening you with guilt and stress, do you smoke illicit drugs? Book in for a health MOT and get your blood pressure and cholesterol checked, and also have a screen for diabetes. Consider which risks you can cut and how much difference that will make.

Risks are real, but reality can be distorted. Think of a particular risk as the number of chances of something happening out of 1000 or 10,000 people, or whatever, rather than a simple percentage. Or compare a particular risk with some other risk you experience every day, to put it in proportion. For example, in Britain travelling to and from a clinic in a car for a vaccination or treatment like the contraceptive pill, is more risky than the vaccination or pill: people have, on average, a one in 8000 chance per year of being in a road accident. That's much more than the chance of being damaged by the treatment.

BE CALCULATING

Using risk charts, like those produced by the European Societies of Cardiology and Hypertension, you can calculate your chance of dying from a heart attack in the next ten years. Get your risk calculated by a doctor, nurse or pharmacist, or if you know your blood pressure or cholesterol level, use the risk charts yourself. There are software programmes that take all health details into account and give you individualised advice (www.medcal.co.uk or www.chdrisk.com). Some stores produce their own healthy living leaflets with lifestyle quizzes – these may alert you to your risks. If you've no actual symptoms of coronary heart disease – as far as you know – then a high risk

Use your appearance, as in IDEA 1, *Appearances aren't always deceptive*, to motivate you.

Try another idea...

is at least a one in five chance of having a heart attack in the next ten years. A low risk is less than a one in twenty chance in that period. You can calculate your risk before and after you manage to reduce your blood pressure or cholesterol or quit smoking – and see the figures plummet.

IN THE BALANCE

You may knowingly have a risky lifestyle or a hobby like scuba-diving (said to have 22 deaths per 100,000 divers a year). You may opt for a treatment you know carries a risk, because you believe the benefits for you outweigh those risks. You need all the facts, and in language you understand, as only you can judge how the exact risks or benefits apply to you. Know the probability of risk and the severity of the potential consequences in order to make an informed decision. People at high risk of stroke from an irregular heartbeat may be advised to take the blood-thinning drug warfarin. But this drug – also a rat poison – can cause a stroke itself, if your blood becomes too thin and you have a bleed in your brain.

'Life's not just being alive, but being well.'
MARTIAL, Roman poet

Defining idea...

How did it go?

Q **Will HRT protect me from getting heart disease if I carry on taking it?**

A *Hormone replacement therapy was thought to protect women against risks of heart disease, and we now know that it doesn't. Around one in a hundred women in their sixties who have taken HRT for at least five years will develop a clot leading to a heart attack or stroke that they wouldn't have had otherwise. But women may still choose HRT for its help with the menopause, feel-good factor and protection against thinning of their bones.*

Q **My doctor says my cholesterol is a bit above normal but not to take statin drugs as I've no other real risk factors. Should I buy statins from a pharmacy or on the internet, anyway, to drive my risks of heart disease down further?**

A *All drugs have side effects. Statins can cause muscle problems, give you headaches, affect your liver function and stir up your gut. Why trigger these if you don't need to? Get all the facts about your risks with and without reducing your cholesterol, so you can decide whether to spend money on a daily statin or on a subscription to your local gym.*

Q **Is it better for me to keep my weight down by smoking as I know my weight will shoot up if I stop?**

A *All risks are relative – and if your parents have heart disease then your relatives are risky for you. Seriously, you've got no choice but to stop smoking and keep your weight down – so make a pledge and keep to it.*

3

New You resolution

Make a 'New You' resolution to be more active. You can't afford to wait for the next new year – that wait could cost you your life. Keeping fit is a must do – for now!

Regular physical activity halves the risk of developing heart disease or having a stroke. And even done after a heart attack, physical activity cuts your risk of then dying by 20%.

It doesn't matter what you do, really – as long as you do something. Here are some ideas.

■ Instead of being a couch potato, get out in the garden and grow your own vegetables. Or pick a new hobby you have always dreamed of doing and make it happen. Switch from long hours spent surfing the internet, to sailing the sea instead. Don't just watch a sport, take part; there are opportunities everywhere. Don't just sit and watch the screen, but take pictures too, walking distances to get just the right shots.

Combining exercising and socialising will make the time you spend getting and staying fit more fun, then you'll be likely to stick with it. What about a regular bike ride with the family? Or link up with a few other cyclists and take it in turns to plan routes for the gang. Take up a regular salsa class or join in a weekly aerobics session; make new friends there, or take your friends along. If you're on a business trip, arrange a round of golf – that'll help with the networking and might clinch a deal, as well as doing you good.

- It's okay to fidget. Every little helps and a little activity is better than none. Keep on the move. Don't sit still for long – get up and fetch that cup of tea or pen. Swing your legs when you're sitting down and don't worry if it annoys other people, it's good for you. Jig around to background music. Get up and walk about regularly when you're stuck at a computer for hours. Don't slump in a seat after you've been out for a meal; get up and do something – maybe walk home from where you've been rather than take the car.

- Workout and work up a sweat. Find a series of exercises that suit you, and do them for five or ten minutes every morning, to get your heart pumping and stretch your back and legs. Any health guide or magazine will profile their tried and tested exercises. Choose a sequence that feels right for you.

- Monitor your heart rate while you're active. Wear an electronic heart rate monitor on your wrist; go for a waterproof one so you can use it swimming or exercising in water. In healthy people, the maximum heart rate varies with age, being about 200 beats per minute for someone who's twenty-five, falling to around 170 beats per minute at sixty-five. The experts recommend that you should exert yourself for twenty to thirty minutes three or more times a week, achieving a heart rate that is at least at 60% of your maximal heart rate, in order to get a training effect. A safe upper limit is to restrict your heart rate to no more than 90% of your maximum, aiming for 65–85% of your maximum when exercising.

If your blood pressure is really high then exercise is contraindicated. Look at IDEA 15, *Get it down*, to find out what you can do to reduce it.

Try another idea...

■ Join a club. You don't have to go to a gym or play sports or use special equipment, but you'll get lots of activity done this way. You'll want to get your money's worth from your gym membership or club fees, and that may help motivate you to keep going regularly. Take advantage of the personal trainer or coach at your gym or club. If you've got a training plan and someone monitoring your progress you'll go far.

■ Choose the right shoes and clothes for your activity so you can walk, run and move without doing yourself harm. Cycling is a fantastic exercise but you need the right saddle on your bike – it carries up to 60% of a cyclist's weight. It's best to choose one filled with gel; that reduces pressure on your genital area. In addition, sit upright as often as you can and lift yourself off the saddle every ten minutes or so.

'The important thing to remember is that this is not a new form of life. It is just a new activity.'
ESTHER DYSON, US journalist

Defining idea...

How did it go?

Q **I've not done any exercise for ages and, though I say it myself, I'm unfit. Do I need to be certified fit by a doctor before I start exercising?**

A *You don't need a certificate, as such, from a doctor. No doctor can confirm with 100% certainty that you'll suffer no health problems from exercise. Even if you press them, they won't guarantee your fitness or they'd be liable if you did have a problem. Do see your doctor if anyone in your immediate family has died suddenly under the age of forty, in case you've a genetic problem of which you're unaware. If you've a fast heart rate at rest (e.g. 120 beats per minute), a heart arrhythmia, or a chronic heart or blood pressure problem, you should seek your doctor's advice before starting to exercise.*

Q **I'd like to do more exercise but I've got angina. Have you any tips for me?**

A *Sure. Warm up slowly. You could try spraying glyceryl trinitrin under your tongue before you start doing any activity to ward off the angina. Wearing a heart rate monitor could mean that you'd be able to stop or slow the activity you were doing when it registered five beats per minute less than the rate that usually triggers your angina. Stop immediately if you develop chest pain, palpitations, undue breathlessness or faintness.*

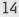

4
Stay bright

You've got a lot to look forward to. So don't look backwards on past misfortunes, but dwell on the happy times in your past. And don't forget to keep your eyes forward on where you're going – otherwise you might step in something horrible...

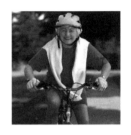

Do you make what you've got count, or do you brood on what's missing? Be optimistic and look on the bright side of life if you want to be happy — and make your heart last longer.

- Try to look at the positive side of things, then, when that cloud drifts across your horizon. It could be that this is the very cloud which stops you getting burnt. For instance, finding out that your cholesterol's high gives you a chance to do something about it, and get the level down by altering your diet or taking statin drugs. It would have been worse to have gone on for years eating fatty foods not knowing that your high cholesterol level was damaging your arteries.

Here's an idea for you...

Think about what you find most rewarding at work. One of the enormous but unspoken realities of life is that most people are basically bored by their jobs. What you value most will probably be to do with your achievements, others recognising your good work, feeling a sense of responsibility or ownership for your work, seeing your career advance and realising that you're growing as a person. Once you know what motivates you, check the extent to which these things are part of your current job. If there's little match, start scanning those job ads now.

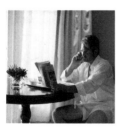

- Craft your life and work so that you can be optimistic. If you're surrounded by misery, it's going to rub off on you so that you feel down too. If you've got a job that makes you stressed and unhappy, then think about changing it. Being part of a happy and close family will make your heart sing; being isolated and friendless will make you miserable. This all affects the state of your heart, so a loving family and good work colleagues are enough to keep the blues away even on the darkest January morning. If you value the company of other people and are interested in what others are doing, you'll rarely get depressed.

- Now, you may sometimes find yourself looking at things in a bleak manner, when your troubles or health problems seem never-ending. Constantly repeating negative thoughts to yourself will make you feel really frustrated about what you're not doing or receiving. Instead, make yourself use positive self-talk inside your head, or to other people. Change negative words and statements into positive ones.

Thanks for buying one of our books! If you'd like to be placed on our mailing list to receive more information on forthcoming releases in the **52 Brilliant Ideas** series just send an e-mail to *info@infideas.com* with your name and address or simply fill in the details below and pop this card in the post. No postage is needed. We promise we won't do silly things like bombard you with lots of junk mail, nor would we even consider letting third parties look at your details. Ever.

Name:..

Address:..

....

e-mail:..

Which book did you purchase?...............................

....

Tell us what you thought of this book and our series; check out the 'Brilliant Communication' bit on the other side of this card.

I am interested in the following subjects:

☐ Health & relationships
☐ Lifestyle & leisure
☐ Arts, literature and music

☐ Careers, finance & personal development
☐ Sports, hobbies & games
☐ Actually, I'd be quite interested in:...........................

And just to say thanks, every month we'll pick 3 random names from a hat (ok, it may be some other cylindrical device) and send a complimentary book from the series. It could be you. So please tell us what book you'd like:...(check out www.52brilliantideas.com for a full list of our titles, or if you prefer we can choose one for you based on your subject interest).

You can change your life with brilliant ideas.

We're passionate about the effect our books have and we have designed them so that they can become an inspiring part of your daily routine. Our books help people to grow, giving them the confidence to believe in themselves and to transform their lives. Every day, around the world, people are regaining control of their lives with our brilliant ideas.

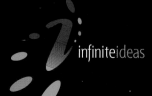
infiniteideas

www.52brilliantideas.com

BrilliantCommunication

- If you enjoyed this book and find yourself cuddling it at night, please tell us. If you think this book isn't fit to use as kindling, please let us know. We value your thoughts and need your honest feedback. We know if we listen to you we'll get it right. Why not send us an e-mail at *listeners@infideas.com*.

- Do you have a brilliant idea of your own that our author has missed? E-mail us at *yourauthor missedatrick@infideas.com* and if it makes it into print in a future edition or appears on our web site we'll send you four books of your choice OR the cash equivalent. You'll be fully credited (if you want) so that everyone knows you've had a brilliant idea.

- Finally, if you've enjoyed one of our books why not become an **Infinite Ideas Ambassador**. Simply e-mail ten of your friends enlightening them about the virtues of the **52 Brilliant Ideas** series and dishing out our web address: www.52brilliantideas.com. Make sure you copy us in at *ambassador@infideas.com*. We promise we won't contact them unless they contact us, but we'll send you a free book of your choice for every ten friends you email. Help spread the word!

■ Look for the humour in a situation whenever you can and enjoy life. Use positive body language, so that you open your arms showing the palms of your hands; maintain eye contact with other people and have a welcoming smile, no matter what. This will cheer you up too.

Look at IDEA 28, *Work at it*, to think more about having a job that motivates you, when you'll cheerfully jump out of bed on an icy cold morning, expecting it to be a good day.

Try another idea...

■ Plan for a rosy retirement, decades before you actually do retire. Then you've got lots to look forward to. You'll want to stay fit and mobile so you can make the most of your free time as you get older, after all. Sounds great, can't wait? Well, can you retire early or work part-time so you've got more leisure to enjoy yourself now?

■ Are you a striker or a goalkeeper? Set goals to win through and appreciate your achievements. You may not turn a cartwheel every time you get a goal, or get a hug from David Beckham, but getting that goal makes the rest of the time spent messing about in the field, or being offside or being tackled by all and sundry, pale into insignificance. So play to your strengths. Set out your plans and targets with your family or your partner, or at work with your boss or colleagues. Then you'll have something to strive for and be optimistic about.

'The optimist proclaims that we live in the best of all possible worlds; and the pessimist fears this is true.'
JAMES BRANCH CABELL, writer

Defining idea...

How did it go?

Q How can I be optimistic when I'm just coming out of my second failed marriage and all my relationships seem doomed?

A *Seek out a partner with a happy-go-lucky nature, who always looks on the bright side. You don't want to be with someone who always expects things to go wrong; you sound as if you've enough negative vibes for two! If you have a new partner with a sunny personality, then some of their approach to life will rub off on you. So get out and meet new people. Do something to shake off your blues – go for a walk, jump in the car, have a bite to eat or a cup of coffee somewhere, or do some voluntary work and help others.*

Q I've been to the doctor and I'm on statin drugs to get my cholesterol down because I've got at least a 30% chance of dying from a heart attack or stroke in the next ten years. There's not much hope for me living to a ripe old age then, is there?

A *There's every hope. Now you're taking statins that will bring your risk of dying right down. So you've probably got at least a 90% chance of still being alive in ten years' time. Think of it like that. Sounds like your odds have improved!*

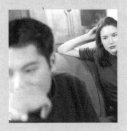 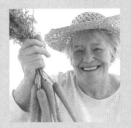

5

Step outside

Put your heart and soles into getting fit. Run a mile – and not away from your fitness challenge, but going for it.

Just thirty minutes spent walking on most days is all it takes for your heart and lungs to be more efficient and healthy, whoever or whatever you are.

Sounds great – and really possible! So here are some ideas about increasing the amount you walk.

You don't have to run a marathon. Walking a half-marathon will be fine – perhaps doing the distance (20 km or 13 miles) over four or five days. Get some comfortable shoes so you've no excuse to stop exercising because of sore feet or tired ankles. Try for that thirty minutes of exercise a day on most days, and this should be brisk exercise that leaves you feeling slightly warm and a bit out of breath: it brings extra benefits to your cardiovascular and metabolic systems. You'll fit this much exercise into your day more easily if you do three blocks of walking for ten-minute bursts at a time, and don't worry – that's just as good as doing it all at once.

Aim for 10,000 steps a day (an average office day takes about 3,000 steps). Use every minute: run errands, make tea for colleagues, whatever. Get a pedometer to count how many steps you actually do. Wear it all day long: when you're walking to work, at work, gardening or dancing. Pedometers are quite cheap and some convert the energy you're using on your steps into the calories you're burning up. If you're a bit of a fidget they may wrongly class movements as steps – so if that's you, you're better clipping your pedometer on and off your belt.

Defining idea...

'I've already set myself a target time. I'm going for less than eleven and a half days.'
JO BRAND, UK comedian, before running a marathon

Build up: gradually walk further or for longer, or increase your speed. Once you've mastered walking on the flat, choose walks that go up and down hills for an extra stretch.

Variety is the price of life. There are lots of activities to choose from to help you integrate more walking into your life, and they're simple ones. What about taking the stairs instead of a lift or escalator (and every time – not just when you feel like it)? To start with, ride on the escalator but start walking half way up, then build up to walking the whole length. Get off the bus one or two stops earlier than normal and walk on. Try leaving the car at home when you don't need to carry heavy bags and walk instead. In fact, get a rucksack so that you can walk and carry anything you need – say, your paperwork to and from the office – easily. And just think – carrying that load of papers on your back will help you to get fit, too. And the great thing is, you don't need to be a sporty person to walk. Everyone's doing it – whether they're a man or woman, fat or thin, old or young, rich or poor. You can walk on your own or in a group, and there are walking groups everywhere. How about joining a local one?

In fact, do more of everything yourself; don't stop at taking specific walks. If you employ a cleaner or gardener, then stop. Digging the garden, mowing the grass or vacuuming the floor are all excellent exercises. Walk to speak to someone in another office instead of phoning or emailing them. Count the steps you're taking while you're doing these things. Maybe stop newspapers being delivered to your door and walk to fetch them instead. You won't have time to read newspapers every day, anyway, now that you're fitting more walking into your life!

Having a dog to exercise will encourage you to go outdoors for a walk or run every day, whatever the weather; check out IDEA 36, *Pet theories*.

Try another idea...

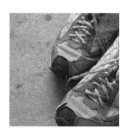 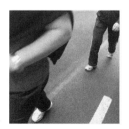

'Keep right on to the end of the road, keep right on to the end, Tho' the way be long, let your heart be strong...'
HARRY LAUDER, singer

Defining idea...

How did it go?

Q How can I exercise when I've got two young children and I'm stuck at home looking after them?

A   *You could push them out in a pram, one in the pram and one sitting on it. Take them to feed the ducks or for a swing in the park. Get into the habit of walking somewhere every single day. Find lots of excuses for short walks – to the shops, to buy the paper, post letters – and leave the car at home. Change your pace, walk quickly and then go slower, so you can cover more distance.*

Q I am so busy with working full time, looking after the house and kids; I don't have time for myself, let alone for any exercise. How can I keep my promises to myself?

A   *Write down those promises and draw up your goals for exercise for the next few weeks. Keep an activity diary; record any activity or type of exercise you do, how long you were active for and how energetic you were. Note down the things that prevented you from carrying out your goals, then try to anticipate these barriers and develop plans in advance of them happening, so you can find ways to avoid them from stopping you becoming more active.*

Q What type of health benefits do I get from brisk walking?

A   *All sorts. You'll lower your cholesterol, bring your blood pressure down a bit and improve the overall condition of your heart and lungs, and strengthen the muscle groups of your legs and bottom. So brisk walking reduces your risk of heart disease, stroke, diabetes and cancer all in one.*

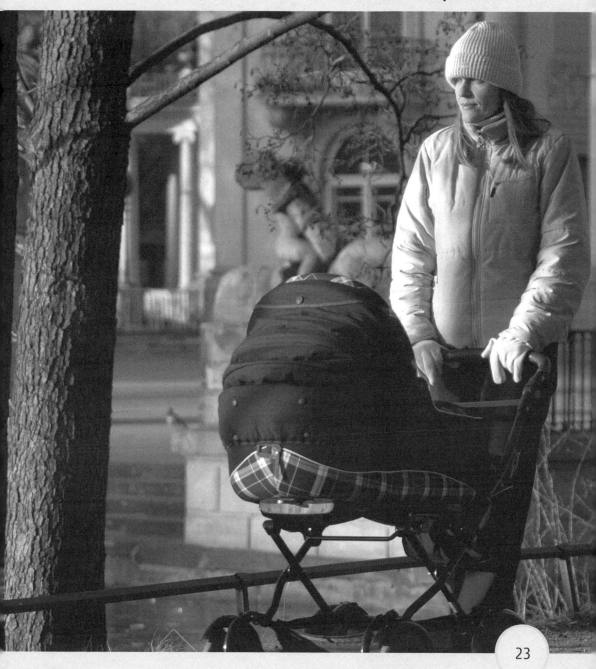

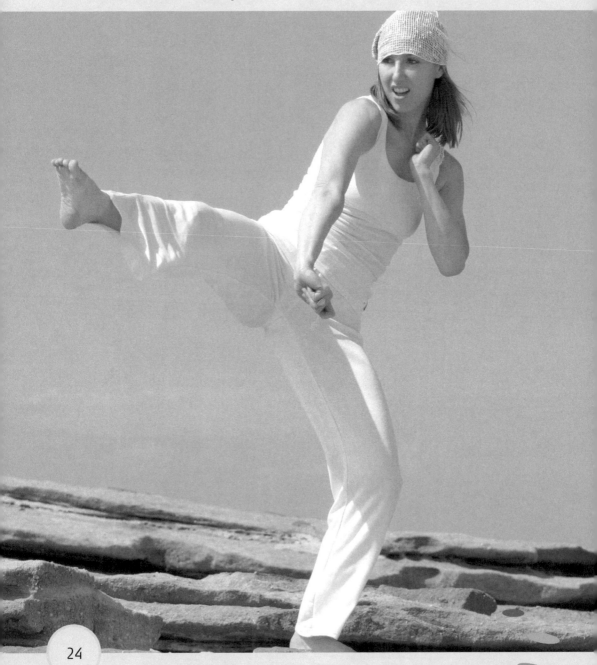

6

Kick-start your exercise

Physical exercise is the antidote to pressures in your life. So muscle into the local walking group, dip into swimming, tire yourself out cycling...

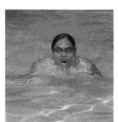

Regular exercise will make you feel better and lift your mood. It'll drop your cholesterol, help prevent your blood clotting, stop high blood pressure from developing and help you maintain a healthy weight.

And, if that's not enough to motivate you: a third and more of coronary heart disease is due to inactivity...

So gradually increase the amount of exercise you do each day. Take your time building up your muscles and ligaments to increase your fitness and their strength. Work towards doing thirty minutes of moderate intensity activity on at least five days a week. The thirty minutes can be accumulated throughout the day in ten- to fifteen-minute bouts. 'Moderate intensity' means breathing slightly harder than normal but staying within your comfort zone. Extend some of your exercise sessions to forty-five minutes or more. This will encourage your body to use some of your fat stores as a source of energy. We're not all born-again athletes. But we can all

Here's an idea for you...

Know your calorie equivalents to exercise. Different types of exercise burn calories at various rates. Cycling at 16 kilometres or 10 miles an hour, for one hour, burns 240 calories. If you pedal really fast at an average 17 mph you'll burn 720 calories in an hour. Walking 5 km in an hour burns off 260 calories; running 9 km in an hour is equivalent to 600 calories. Cross-country skiing really devours calories – 1400 per hour. Compare these to just standing about, when you'll burn a mere 100 calories an hour.

Defining idea...

'Every day, in every way, I am getting better and better.'
ÉMILE COUÉ, French psychotherapist

integrate exercise into our day, however busy we are. Here's how. Start when you get up in the morning. No, not with a 'Jane Fonda' type of workout, unless you want to, but more of a marching on the spot while you brush your teeth, or loosening your shoulders and stretching your limbs when drying off after your morning shower or as you get dressed. Exercise your pelvic floor or move your lumbar spine around when sitting in the car or on the bus or tube. Squeeze in various muscle groups and hold for the count of ten. Here are some more ideas.

■ Walk up and down stairs, pointedly avoiding the lift or escalator. All the better if you're carrying heavy bags – that's extra exercise without you realising it, except the huffing and puffing and sweat lines on your clothes are a bit of a giveaway. And start campaigning for extra provision for bicycles: then capture some of the energy you put into that campaign for when you're actually cycling!

■ Get up from your desk little and often. Take frequent trips to the printer and photocopier. Do exercises while you're waiting for a printout or the kettle to boil – maybe some dance steps if no one's looking...

■ Remember when people actually took a lunch break? Well, get out the staff charter, if you have one, rediscover your entitlement, and get out there – for a walk, a quick swim or cycle ride. Go for a purpose if that helps, perhaps to post a letter, buy your sandwiches or debrief with a friend.

■ Do some exercise when you're watching TV – don't just sit there, slumped, doing an imitation of a corpse. Pause the video and take a walking break. A quick spin on your exercise bike or ten sit-ups, while watching your programme or in the commercial break, and you've done some of your exercise stint for the day.

■ Do your own housework or gardening; treasure the opportunity to work off those calories or strengthen your muscles. Spend the money you've saved on domestic help on gym membership or new running shoes.

■ Rediscover dancing. Insure your feet, if you're a beginner, against breakages. Take plenty of plasters for all those blisters.

Any exercise helps. If you're on the move and it's keeping you warm, then it's good for you. The best activities for boosting your weight loss and fitness are those involving large muscle groups. These are mainly aerobic exercises: walking, running, swimming or cycling.

Walking is one of the best forms of exercise and it's free – unless you're on an expensive walking holiday somewhere exotic. Hot foot it to IDEA 5, *Step outside*, for more.

Try another idea...

'My heart is in my boots.'
BORIS JOHNSON, UK politician

Defining idea...

27

How did it go?

Q   **I'm keen on weightlifting. Could lifting those heavy weights put too much strain on my heart muscles?**

A   *The thing about weightlifting is that you take a big breath and hold it – and, all told, this exercise puts your blood pressure up which is bad for your heart. Lift a lesser weight many times, rather than a heavy weight less frequently.*

Q   **What's the best form of exercise for someone who's really overweight like me?**

A   *One of the few advantages of being overweight is that you use more energy when you're walking than a slimmer person does. You won't carry on with regular exercise unless you enjoy doing it, though – or unless you're a masochist. So go for exercise that fits your lifestyle, and one you like doing. When exercise is a pleasure, fitness is easy.*

Q   **How can you prioritise yourself over the kids after you've been out at work all day and not seen much of them?**

A   *It's never too early to teach your children good habits and ensure that they're active too. Can you exercise together more, having fun as a family? For example, you could swim while the children have their swimming lessons. Choose activity holidays which can involve you all; use the gym at times when all ages are welcome or go to one where there's a crèche.*

7

What's in your fridge?

Take a good look at all the food and drink stored in your fridge. What you've got in there is at the heart of what you eat.

The contents of your fridge say a lot about your health and how much you're trying for a healthy lifestyle. Do a snap check and have a look in yours soon after you've done your weekly shop...

WHAT'S INSIDE?

When you look in your fridge, is there plenty of fruit and vegetables? If you're going to have at least five portions a day, which you should do in order to keep fit and well, you're going to find fruit juice and at least some fruit and veg there, even if you've a laden fruit bowl on the side. Perhaps there are some juicy grapefruit, enough for a half or whole one for every breakfast for the rest of the week. There should be plenty of salad – enough for some every day. As a starter, salad helps to curb your appetite so that you consume fewer calories during the rest of the meal: and, of course, it counts as one of your five portions, and don't forget to use fat-free salad dressing or low-fat mayonnaise, as well. The fat content of any prepared

Here's an idea for you...

Keep a great variety of foods for making packed lunches in the fridge. Taking your lunch to work with you will help to reduce temptation – no chips or burgers for you from the canteen, or fattening sandwiches. Instead, perhaps, healthy strips of lean ham, or pieces of tuna with a salad, or crispbread, all accompanied by fruit, yoghurt, a light cheese spread and bread sticks...

potato salads or coleslaw will be telling. There's a range of health difference between standard varieties and those that are low fat – and watch the sugar content, too.

Then you'd expect to see some dairy products and lean meat, eggs and some fish, semi-skimmed or skimmed milk for cereal and drinks. The presence of double cream or full-fat crème fraîche will be a dead giveaway to your bad habits. If they're there you don't really mean all those pledges about low-cholesterol foods, do you? Even if you got it in for guests, shouldn't you have chucked what was left down the sink when you washed up the dinner plates? There should also be half-fat cheese, but not too much of it. Yoghurts are good for you, if they're the low-fat kind that isn't stuffed with sugar. Any butter? Well, that would get me hunting for the thick slices of bread I'd be tempted to plaster it on... Spreads should be plant sterols and sunflower oil or the equivalent, to bring down your cholesterol, and vegetable oil sprays minimise the oil you use for cooking. Look in the freezer compartment for the hidden, naughty-but-nice foods: ice cream, standby bread and cakes. Was the special two-for-one offer too good to miss – are there loads of pastries and ready meals in there?

Now, what about meat? It's OK if there's bacon, but hopefully that will be just a few lean rashers and not the streaky kind. A fridge stacked with meat would be worrying, because people who eat a diet with mainly vegetable protein rather than animal protein are 30% less likely to die of heart disease. Finally, there'll be no heavy puddings, hopefully. After all, there's no need if you've got delicious fruit and yoghurts stored in your fridge.

Get your children started with good habits by keeping healthy snacks and drinks for them in the fridge. Check out IDEA 42, *Don't kid yourself*, for more cool ideas for kids.

Try another idea...

WHAT'LL YOU HAVE?

When the door of the fridge swung open, was there a clink of bottles or the quiet chug of unsweetened fruit juice in its carton? If you find half a dozen bottles of wine or beer it's difficult to believe that you're keeping to the recommended weekly units of alcohol, or are all those bottles being chilled on the off-chance that a group of thirsty friends might suddenly descend on you unexpectedly? Is there a good selection of low-calorie drinks? Even a nice cold jug of tap water will appeal, waiting there for you after a hard day at work.

HOME-MADE...

It's really great if there's evidence of home-cooked meals. Hopefully there'll be a vegetarian dish full of peas, lentils or beans, or maybe a casserole of fish or lean meat. And with any gravy made from home-made stock: if there's any fat in it, it can be easily scraped off before the casserole is reheated, as it will have solidified in the fridge. A batch of home-made soup will score highly, so long as there's barely a trace of salt in it and the flavour's been enhanced by herbs – so no need for salt at the table.

'It's a great thing to know our vices.'
CICERO

Defining idea...

31

How did it go?

Q   I'm a naughty nibbler – so what should I have in my fridge?

A   *Go for some pre-prepared packs of sticks of carrots or chunks of cucumber or spring onion. Keep them in an airtight container so they stay crispy and moist. Buy one or two fridge magnets with healthy messages on them or rude reminders about overeating.*

Q   What are the best kind of ready meals for when I come in from a hard day at the office, to heat up for the family?

A   *Make up your own to store in your fridge or freezer. Prepare a job lot at the weekend or when you've got the time. Cook several times as much as you need of very healthy meals, containing little fat or salt. Eat one meal fresh and freeze or cool the rest, depending on how much you've made and when you're going to eat it. Label everything clearly so you know what it is, how many portions are included and when you prepared it.*

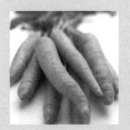 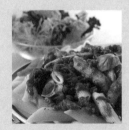

8

Food for thought

Here's some food for thought. Veto salt, increase your fruit and veg intake, replace fat with carbohydrate and you cut your chances of heart disease. Simple as that.

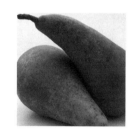

Eating well does not mean affording rich food...

It means eating healthily so your normal weight reduces strain on your heart, keeps your cholesterol and blood pressure down, and prevents fatty deposits or clots forming in your bloodstream. Go for a cardio-friendly diet.

- Fat has over twice as many calories as a portion of starch or protein weighing the same, so reduce the amount you eat. Beware of invisible fats such as those which occur in foods like biscuits, cakes, chocolate, pastry and savoury snacks; always read the labels. Trim fat from meat and poultry. Opt for low-fat milk, dairy products and spreads. Choose to bake or grill rather than fry (even use oven chips instead of fried potatoes). Fill up on bread, cereals, potatoes, fruit and vegetables. Choose low-fat snacks to suit your taste; everyone has their own favourites. Then you should also try and avoid salt on those snacks, or on any other foods, as far as possible to keep your blood pressure down. People with

Here's an idea for you... **Lots of oily fish is good for you, which may seem surprising. That's sardines, salmon, pilchards, mackerel, herring or tuna. The oil in fish seems to help reduce the risk or the severity of heart disease by lowering the fats in your bloodstream, making your blood cells less sticky. Eat oily fish two or three times a week if you can, or at least once a week to ward off heart disease; even eating fish just three times a month seems to make a difference. This shouldn't be fried fish or fish cooked in batter – you'll undo the good from the fish with the fat that accompanies it – so look up some mouth-watering recipes for cooking fish that don't involve frying.**

healthy hearts tend to eat more wholegrain and high-fibre foods; rice bran, for instance, is brilliant and it lowers cholesterol.

■ Grow your own. Go back to nature and grow your own fruit and vegetables wherever you can, in a back garden or yard. If they're just waiting to be picked, you'll eat more. And actually growing them will keep you more active, which all helps your heart too. Or you could go to farmers' markets and food cooperatives for some really fresh produce.

■ Eating at least five portions a day of fruit and vegetables could cut deaths from heart disease, stroke and cancer by a fifth. Just one more portion of fruit and veg a day will lower your risk of heart disease by 4% and cut your risk of stroke by 6%. The potassium in fruit and veg is thought to help keep your blood pressure down and steady the rhythm of your heart. A glass of fruit juice counts as one portion, and the fruit and veg can be fresh, raw or cooked, tinned or frozen. To measure one portion of berries or grapes you'll need a cupful; for small individual fruit, like plums, eat two; for dried fruit take a tablespoonful – and for bigger fruit like apples and bananas eat a whole one. Sorry, but you can't count potatoes when you're tallying up your five portions a day; they don't seem to share the same heart disease prevention properties as other vegetables; they're a good source of starch, though. And be careful with avocados – they might be a fruit, but they're full of fat…

Have a polymeal once a day: see IDEA 10, *Designer polymeal*, for an explanation. Experts reckon it'll cut your chances of heart disease by three-quarters.

Try another idea…

■ You'll help your kids' hearts, too, by starting them on good eating habits early in life. They'll learn from having you as a good role model, and get a taste for healthy food at the same time. You'll be investing in their health, not making fatty deposits in their blood.

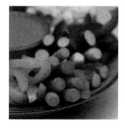

'I eat to live, to serve, and also, if it so happens, to enjoy, but I do not eat for the sake of enjoyment.'
MAHATMA GANDHI

Defining idea…

How did it go?

Q **We had chips with everything in my family. Now I've set up on my own I want to eat more healthily. Where do I start?**

A *What about finding a holiday with a course in healthy cooking? You could have fun in the sun and learn a lot. Buy or borrow recipe books – there are loads on the market by health gurus – or start a scrapbook and cut out tasty tips from newspapers and magazines. Get a stock of herbs and other healthy ingredients which will give your meals a zing.*

Q **I've eaten a rubbish diet for years. Is there any point changing now I'm middle-aged?**

A *It's never too late to watch what you eat. A healthy diet will increase your chances of surviving a heart attack. It'll reduce the risks of you developing heart disease and high blood pressure in the first place, and slow the damage if you've already got heart problems. It'll be much less likely that one of your coronary arteries will become blocked by a blood clot. Go for it.*

Q **Can you give me some advice about quick and easy meals that are healthy too?**

A *Well, avoid any ready meals from supermarkets unless you've read the labels and are sure that the fat and salt content is low enough to be fine. Fish and lean meat dishes with salad or veg are going to be a healthy choice. Bulk up a casserole with lots of vegetables. Microwaving needs no extra fat or oil and is quick to do – an easy win for you.*

9

Keep circulating

Fur keeps animals warm and it's better left to them. You don't want fur coating the arteries in your legs or heart or your brain where it can cause poor circulation, a heart attack, stroke or mini-stroke.

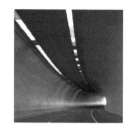

Lowering cholesterol saves lives — and that could be your life, after all.

You can partly control your cholesterol by eating a healthy diet containing only a little saturated fat and lots of fibre so it's less likely that cholesterol will be absorbed into your bloodstream.

Cholesterol is a fatty substance which is mainly made in the liver from saturated fats in food. Cholesterol is carried round your bloodstream by proteins. Together cholesterol and proteins are called lipoproteins. There's also a group of fatty substances called triglycerides. The lipoproteins have two components: high density lipoprotein (HDL) and low density lipoprotein (LDL). Think back to your childhood when you played at being 'goodies' and 'baddies'. The HDL or 'good' cholesterol removes cholesterol from circulating in the blood and protects you against heart

Here's an idea for you...

Almost anyone with an increased risk of heart disease is recommended to take a drug to lower their cholesterol, whether their baseline cholesterol is at a normal level or not. Ask your pharmacist or health care worker if you should start treatment if you're not on such a drug already. Statins are the most commonly used treatments and work by reducing the amount of bad LDL cholesterol in your bloodstream. They can reduce total cholesterol levels by more than 20%. Take them in the evening as most of your cholesterol is made at night.

disease. The LDL or 'bad' cholesterol gets taken up by the walls lining the arteries in your heart. So you want a low level of LDL and a high level of HDL to protect you against heart disease and avoid the furring up of your arteries. However, genetics also play a part in fixing your cholesterol level. With the best possible diet, you can only reduce your total cholesterol by 5–10%. But if you reduce your cholesterol by 1% you'll lower your risk of developing heart disease by about 2%. Your aim is to have a cholesterol level less than 5mmol/litre. Here's some more necessary information.

Monounsaturated fats help reduce the bad LDL level but not the good or protective HDL. They're found in olive oil, walnut oil, rapeseed oil and avocado. Some margarines and spreads are made from this type of fat. Polyunsaturated fats help lower the LDL too, but also the HDL, unfortunately. They're found in cornflower oil, sunflower oil, soya oil and fish oil. Some margarines and spreads are made from these type of fats. Omega-3 fats are polyunsaturated fats that help lower your triglyceride level and prevent your blood from clotting. They're found in oily fish and fish oil. Your body can manufacture the same omega-3 fats from the oil in walnuts, soya and rapeseed.

Now, whatever you do, avoid saturated fats. They increase LDL levels. You'll find them in butter, hard cheese, suet, ghee, coconut oil and lard, full-fat dairy products, cakes, biscuits, pastries and savoury snacks. Replace any saturated fats in your diet with small amounts of the unsaturated types and omega-3 oils. Overall, reduce the total amount of fat that you eat, especially if you're overweight. About a third of the calories in your diet should come from fat, and less than 10% of those from saturated fat.

Eating more fibre can help; check out the healthy diet described in IDEA 8, *Food for thought*, for more ideas.

Try another idea...

Eating at least five portions a day of fruit and vegetables cuts the chances of dying from heart disease, stroke and cancer by a fifth. The vitamins and other substances, called antioxidants, in the fruit and veg is probably what does the good. Without oxidation, cholesterol does not form the fatty deposits that cause harm by lining the walls of your arteries. This can't be the whole story, though, as just taking vitamin supplements without eating the fruit and veg doesn't have the same effects. Cranberry juice is good for your heart as well. A glass of cranberry juice a day can boost your body's supply of good cholesterol or HDL considerably.

'As I see it, every day you do two things: build health or produce disease in yourself.'
ADELLE DAVIS, American health authority

Defining idea...

Q   Are all foods labelled 'low fat' OK?

A   *Foods labelled as low fat are not always so. They may be lower than other, similar foods without a low-fat tag, but might be a lot higher in fat than other foods. For instance, low-fat pâté still has plenty of fat in it compared to lean cooked ham.*

Q   Any tips on how best to limit fat when I'm eating out?

A   *You can only be really sure what fat is in your meals when you've prepared them yourself. You could ask for half a portion of meat for a main meal, and extra vegetables or salad, or make a starter do for your main course in order to cut the volume. Bread sticks make good nibbles. Choose thin pizza bases and sprinkle a little parmesan on for a strong taste without much fat. Go for stir-fried instead of deep-fried dishes. Choose boiled rice rather than egg-fried rice, pilau or biryani rice, noodles or any creamy sauce. With Indian food, the drier tandoori and bhuna dishes are less fatty than creamy ones like korma or masala. And do be aware that Indian food may be cooked in ghee – clarified butter.*

Q   Can I tell if my cholesterol is high or must I have a blood test?

A   *There are few noticeable symptoms. So if you've any other risk factors for heart disease, like being overweight or smoking, have a test.*

10

Designer polymeal

Design your ideal polymeal. It's not the latest celebrity diet, it's about putting together the right ingredients to reduce your risk of heart disease and protect you from the furring up of your arteries.

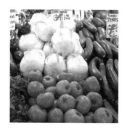

Eating fish, dark chocolate, fruit, vegetables, almonds and garlic, and drinking wine can lower your risks of getting heart disease, or make it less serious. But you have to combine these foods in the right way.

NOT TOO MUCH OF A GOOD THING

To reduce your risk by the maximum possible you should have the following quantities of the recommended food and drink (though you might need to consider weight gain!): 150 ml of wine per day, 114 g of fish four times a week, 100 g of dark chocolate a day; 400 g of fruit and vegetables daily, 2.7 g of fresh garlic (or the equivalent 900 mg of dried garlic) every day, and 68 g of almonds each day. Now, this kind of food can reduce your risk of heart disease by a staggering three-quarters

Here's an idea for you...

Instead of constructing a polymeal that contains all the health-giving ingredients at one time, go for a polydiet and integrate all the ingredients into your usual everyday foods. So add chopped almonds to your cereal packet: pour them in and shake the packet up, so you'll be eating them everyday. Add almonds everywhere – you can sprinkle them on salads, add them to yoghurt and curries. Buy plenty of fish and then experiment with steaming it, baking it or low-fat frying it; freeze it for other days. Learn to handle garlic, by crushing or chopping it with salt, microwaving it to soften it, even bashing the clove with the side of a knife to get the skin off. Melt dark chocolate in your microwave and add various chopped fruits. Make a hot chocolate drink with dark chocolate, milk and honey...

and it shows how much you can do for yourself if you've got a taste for it. Translate these benefits into effects on your life expectancy, and you'd expect to live an extra six or seven years! Let's look at some different kinds of polymeal to give you an idea of how you can use the information.

FRENCH POLYMEAL

For starters, try raw salmon marinated in lemon juice with lettuce, tomato and kiwi slices with olive and canola oil, garlic and balsamic vinegar. For the main course have fresh roasted cod with garlic seasoning, surrounded with tomato and potato slices and spinach leaves. Finish off with chocolate cake with almonds. Wash the meal down with a white Bordeaux wine. This menu is rich in omega-3 polyunsaturated fatty acids, reputed to prevent dementia, so it might have other health benefits too.

POSH POLYMEAL

Prepare warm chilli crab cakes in a fresh garlic dressing for your starter, with salad leaves and fine green and red pepper slices. Go on to a main course of trout with an almond crust, poached in red wine and accompanied by courgettes in garlic butter, with baby carrot batons, mangetout and new potatoes basted in olive oil. Your dessert will be a rich dark chocolate mousse with fresh strawberries dipped in dark chocolate. Try some dark chocolate petit fours and cream truffles with your (decaffeinated) coffee. Then a glass of red wine...

Look back at IDEA 8, *Food for thought*, to remind yourself about healthy eating and having a balanced diet with plenty of fruit and vegetables.

Try another idea...

A WINNING POLYMEAL

Courgette, pea and chopped leeks in orange sauce with Irish wheaten bread can be your starter for this meal. Follow on with crispy fillet of sea bream with garlic potatoes and a beetroot and onion salad, and with red wine to drink. Then finish with chocolate, almond and raspberry pie.

AUSSIE POLYDAY

Have a fruity breakfast of kiwi fruit, strawberries, apricots, seven almonds and a plain yoghurt. Then a 'vege-rice' lunch consisting of broccoli florets, asparagus spears, three chopped almonds, more steamed vegetables and rice. Dinner is a treat – tuna, flounder or snapper baked in the oven,

'They always say time changes things, but you actually have to change them yourself.'
ANDY WARHOL

Defining idea...

43

smeared with olive oil and garlic. Serve the fish with roast potatoes and a small glass of wine. For pudding, opt for poached pears in a melted chocolate sauce and garnished by almonds.

ROMANTIC POLYMEAL

You'll start off with cherry tomatoes with mozzarella cheese, using fresh basil and olive oil. Go on to eat monkfish with a Mediterranean-style filling – with chopped garlic, rosemary, tomatoes, basil and black olives – maybe wrapped in Parma ham, and served with a selection of vegetables. Choose a banana swathed in a rich chocolate sauce for your desert, garnished with almond slices. You'll be drinking red wine with this meal – 150 ml each. Drink cinnamon-flavoured hot chocolate instead of your usual after-dinner coffee.

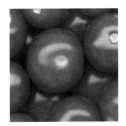
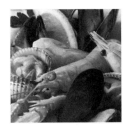

Q   Are there any disadvantages to polymeal eating?

A   Well, you might be one of those people who whiff a bit after eating garlic. And if you don't keep to the amounts of fish suggested you might get raised mercury levels in your blood from eating too much, especially if it's large fish like shark or swordfish. And too much dark chocolate gives you... er... let me see – weight gain. Shame about that.

Q   Some expensive ingredients here, aren't there? What cheaper options can you recommend?

A   Keep it simple and keep it to your taste. The sample menus here just show the versatility of fruit and vegetables, garlic, almonds, fish, dark chocolate and wine, and how they can be combined. Just do it your way, either as a polymeal or scattered throughout the day. Being healthier and living longer has got to be worth the investment. Look at http://bmj.com/cgi/eletters/329/7480/0-f for more meal ideas.

How did it go?

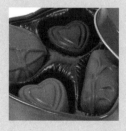 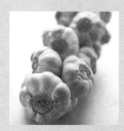

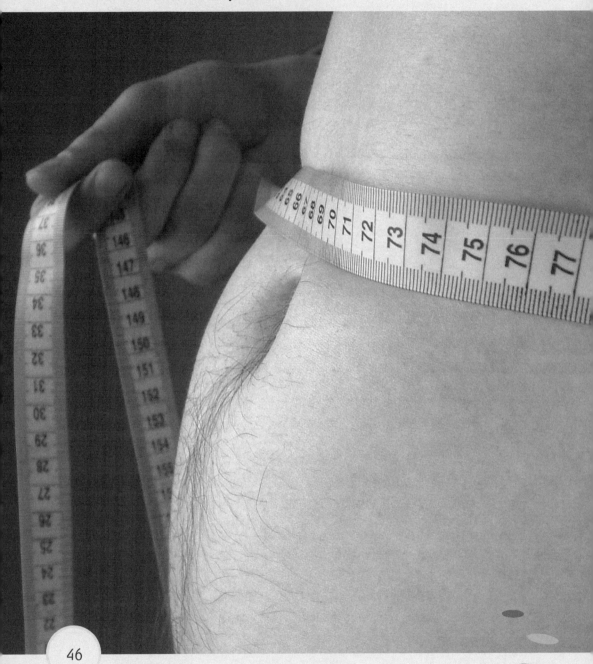

11

Battle of the bulge

Is there a fat chance of you being a normal weight? Think again, and put your heart first, not your stomach, because your weight really matters.

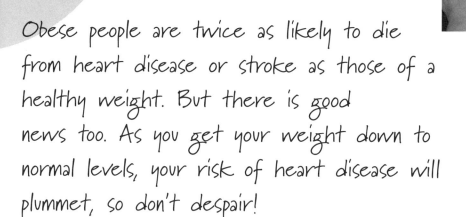

Obese people are twice as likely to die from heart disease or stroke as those of a healthy weight. But there is good news too. As you get your weight down to normal levels, your risk of heart disease will plummet, so don't despair!

There are four approaches you can try. Start by sticking to a sensible diet where the various food groups are well balanced. Then you could change your behaviour: stop snacking between meals, buy rewards and luxuries which aren't food or drink, eat main meals early-ish in the day or join a slimming group. Thirdly, you could take up regular exercise or more sport. Finally, there's medical treatment... a last resort is using a prescribed drug, but you must be truly obese and should have tried at least three months of diet and exercise first. Orlistat works by blocking the way you absorb fat in your gut; at the same time your cholesterol and blood pressure fall, great side effects of this drug. You should lose around 10% of your body weight by

Here's an idea for you...

Are you suffering from portion distortion? Think little, not large when selecting your portion. One person's 'small' portion can be another person's 'medium' or even 'large' portion. It's all in the eye (and stomach, unfortunately) of the beholder. Avoid 'all you can eat' buffets, meal-deal lunches and king-size chocolate bars. Remember what a typical serving looks like: a portion of fish is the size of a chequebook, a medium-sized potato the same size as a standard light bulb, a portion of cooked pasta is the size of a ball of string, and a portion of meat should be the size of a pack of playing cards.

Defining idea...

'Outside every fat man is an even fatter man trying to close in.'
KINGSLEY AMIS, author, *One Fat Englishman*

six months to justify being on it. An absolutely last resort if you're obese is surgery: getting your stomach stapled or guillotined – ouch.

Right, now for some practical tips.

- In general, foods with a high fibre content fill you up for longer, giving you a slow trickle of energy. You don't need to eat just because you're hungry; that's a common mistake. Eat a low-fat diet where fat makes up about only 20–30% of your total calories. Couple that with high-fibre foods like wholegrain bread and pasta.

- Eat slowly, and put your food on small plates – you'll eat less in the long run. Always refuse seconds, and just eat enough to satisfy your appetite. Have a drink of water before a meal so that you partly fill your stomach before starting on the food.

- And always go for low-calorie or calorie-free drinks. Alcohol's high in calories, and that way it won't undermine your resolve to eat little and healthily, either. Alcohol-free beers and wines contain around half the calories of standard drinks. Sip water when you're drinking, too, to make your alcoholic drink last longer. Don't let other people refill your glass, unless you really want it.

- Finally, don't sit it out. Walking a mile uses up 100–150 kilocalories of energy, depending on your body weight. Weigh that against the energy requirements for a moderately active man of 3000 calories a day, or for a woman, 2200 calories. One of the few advantages of being overweight is that you use more energy. Cram exercise into your day so that your energy output balances the amount and type of food you eat. Be creative, not conventional, about exercising: when watching TV do a mini-workout in the ad break instead of fetching more chocolate. If you're working from home, intersperse your day with brisk walks; you'll work better for it. Walk the children to school and back; leave your car at home. You can even enjoy housework – you might savour an hour of window cleaning, thinking of the glass of wine you'll enjoy when you've finished, equivalent to the 160 kilocalories you're working off.

If one of your motivating factors for losing weight is your appearance, then read IDEA 1, *Appearances aren't always deceptive*, for another look at this.

Try another idea...

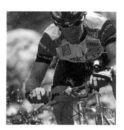

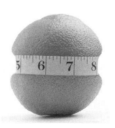

'*My advice if you insist on slimming: eat as much as you like – just don't swallow it.*'
HARRY SECOMBE, comedian

Defining idea...

How did it go?

Q How much extra exercise do I need to do to lose a reasonable amount of weight each week?

A   *To lose one kilo of weight, you need a 7500 kilocalorie deficit, on average. That's the gap between the calories you eat and the energy you need to burn up to keep your body ticking over, and doing activities and movement. So think about how many calories various activities use up, and work out what you would like to do. A daily deficit of just 600 kilocalories will give you a steady weight loss of a kilo a fortnight.*

Q Why do I lose so little weight when I'm on the same diet as my sister, who's really fat and is doing really well?

A   *The more obese you are, the more energy you expend just living, let alone moving about and working (and men use up more calories a day than women, too). A very obese person can lose weight on a diet of 2000 calories a day, whereas someone of more normal build won't. You need a diet crafted for you, and not your sister, taking account of your weight now, and how much energy you burn during the day.*

Q How can I satisfy my hunger so I don't eat as much?

A   *Opt for high fibre foods and ones with a high water content which bulks them up, like fruit and vegetables. Foods that contain chromium such as egg yolk, brewer's yeast and molasses can reduce your hunger pangs. Capsaicin, found in chillies and peppers, can suppress your appetite. Focus on what you're eating and enjoy it but always stop as soon as you're full. One last tip: don't eat in front of the TV; you'll get distracted and might eat lots more than you normally would.*

12

In the kitchen

They say the kitchen's the central hub of the house. It's central to your health too, as it's where you store and cook your food.

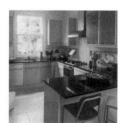

It knows your secrets. You may fool your slimming class instructor or personal trainer, but you can't fool your kitchen...

Equip your kitchen so you can cook up low fat food in healthy ways. Then don't bypass your kitchen via the take-away or snack bar, tempting though it might be.

CUPBOARD LOVE

- You should have healthy foods in store, like high-fibre flour and pasta. Dried fruit is good (eaten in moderation) and so are packs of high-fibre cereals and oatmeal. Your cupboard shouldn't be overflowing with lots of refined foods, like bags of sugar, cake mix or packs of biscuits.

- The type of pans you're using for cooking will dictate how much fat is in your diet. Go for non-stick pans so you don't need to cover the bottom in loads of fat before heating them or frying meat or fish. Though pans for stir-frying do need a little more fat to get them going, it's minimal and the quick cooking method means that most of the vitamins in your vegetables and meat or fish are well

Here's an idea for you...

Your kitchen scales are not just for finding out how heavy your letters and parcels are before stamping and posting. They're there to check the weight of the portions of food you're eating. You might think you know what 200 grams of cheese looks like but you'll probably cut and eat double that unknowingly, or you might think you know what constitutes a portion of the meat or fish that's described in a calorie counter book, but you don't really know until you actually weigh them. A little bit extra could make a big difference, and you could easily – and innocently – be fooling yourself, so don't guess.

preserved. Steamers are also great – there are no hidden calories when you cook up your vegetables or fish in these. Hopefully any roasting tins have got fat-straining racks standing inside them.

■ Gravy boats should have a funnel arrangement to siphon off the fat content of the gravy or sauce when it's been left standing for a while.

■ And, fingers crossed, there'll be no fat fryer. Fat fryers are lethal for your heart. Even when you cook chips or doughnuts in a basket and shake off excess fat, they're still packed with it. So chuck your fat fryer away while you're still alive to do so! And it's not just fat fryers: sandwich cookers need lots of fat wiped on to ensure the sandwich doesn't stick, so by the time you've added in the cheese inside the sandwich, the fat content of your snack will be massive.

WORKTOPS

■ The worktop in your kitchen should be a busy place and show evidence of lots of home cooking: if you cook things yourself you can be sure that only healthy ingredients are inside your casserole or risotto. And perhaps there will be a bowl full to the brim of tantalising fruit for your five-a-day quota. A fruit press or squeezer will be another way to get lots of vitamin C in fresh fruit juice.

Take a quick look in the fridge to check on stocks of fruit and juice, lean meat and low-fat spreads – look at IDEA 7, What's in your fridge?

Try another idea...

- Maybe there's a bread machine, where you make your home-baked bread. That's fine, so long as the bread that emerges from your machine is not over-dense because it's not properly risen. If it is, then you'll end up eating twice as much bulk – and therefore more carbohydrate and calories – than you would compared with commercially prepared bread.

- Look around the kettle area. Is there a range of options for healthy hot drinks? You want to have choices of decaffeinated coffee and tea, maybe low-calorie clear soups. That's probably where the cordials and other cold drinks are too. Look particularly for decaffeinated and no-sugar fizzy drinks; shudder at sweet cordials and squashes, which are just sugar by another name, or drinking chocolate which might persuade you to give in to your chocolate addiction...

- Your microwave has got to be the centrepiece of a healthy kitchen. It's going to let your home-prepared frozen meals spring to life, and save you from resorting to junky ready meals when you're starving and just in from a heavy day's work. And you can cook up food in the microwave without adding fat, so find out how to use yours for cooking, not just for heating things through or defrosting.

'The first step to getting the things you want out of life is this: decide what you want.'
BEN STEIN, US writer and broadcaster

Defining idea...

53

How did it go?

Q **I'm just about to leave home and set up in a bedsit. No kitchen there, then – what'll I do?**

A *A microwave has got to be the answer for you. And start building up a collection of healthy cookery books that you can take with you when you move on to your next flat or house.*

Q **What kinds of cooking equipment can I get to cook up my favourite food – chips, sorry – in a healthy way?**

A *You can microwave chips... But you can also microwave crisps cut from very thinly sliced potato in a special container that looks a bit like a plate rack – try those instead of chips. You could even buy a fat-free hot air fryer so you can have your chips and eat them – this fries, grills and bakes using only the moisture from the food itself, but that would be an expensive answer to your question and the other alternatives are cheaper.*

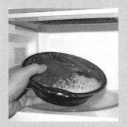
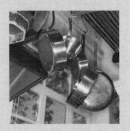

13

Down with homocysteine

There's growing recognition that high levels of homocysteine are associated with heart disease, so watch out for it. Here's some help.

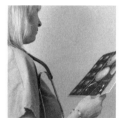

We're still learning a lot about homocysteine. Scientists are trying to establish the facts, but while they do, it's a good idea to pay attention to your homocysteine levels.

Homocysteine is an amino acid normally found in blood. Children with the rare condition, homocystinuria, develop atherosclerosis – a widespread thickening or furring of their arteries with fatty deposits. If they are left untreated they die of complications, having strokes or heart attacks, clots on their lungs or in other blood vessels. When the homocystinuria is treated in ways that lower their homocysteine levels, those children's risks of heart attacks and strokes fall too. So now it's believed that the raised homocysteine level in their bloodstream means that they have an increased risk of having a heart attack, a stroke or having a clot form.

But we don't yet know whether it's the homocysteine itself that's dangerous. We do know that homocysteine generates superoxide and hydrogen peroxide which seem to damage artery walls. Homocysteine also seems to encourage clots to form. It prevents small arteries from dilating, so they're more easily obstructed.

Here's an idea for you... **Why not opt for a Mediterranean diet? That'll have olive oil, grains and cereals, pasta, fruits, vegetables and legumes, limited amounts of eggs and dairy products, some fish and poultry, and even some wine in moderation. When people with high homocysteine levels go for a diet like this – which is high in retinoids, folic acid and fibre – their homocysteine concentration is reduced, and that seems to help prevent them from developing heart disease. An added bonus for your health is that having a high level of folic acid in your diet also protects you against colon cancer and dementia!**

Homocysteine interacts with the low-density lipoprotein component of cholesterol, causing it to stick to artery walls. But there needs to be a lot more evidence about how harmful homocysteine actually is before doctors advocate that people get routinely screened for homocysteine levels, or before they start treatments with vitamin therapy for people with heart disease on a wider scale. It's a case of watch this space, and wait for more research to be published. People with kidney failure, and people who have received organ transplants, seem to have high levels of homocysteine. Indian Asians seem to have higher levels of homocysteine than white Europeans. Black South Africans have lower levels than white South Africans. We still don't know why...

We *do* know that a healthy homocysteine level is less than 12 micromolecules per litre: in one research study, men with a level of over 15 micromolecules per litre were nearly three times more likely to die of heart disease. But, you guessed it, research hasn't yet definitely, absolutely, shown that lowering homocysteine levels reduces your chance of having a heart attack or stroke. In the meantime, it clearly pays to keep your homocysteine levels down. It is thought to be good to have plenty of folic acid in your diet – this can help to lower your homocysteine levels.

Go to IDEA 10, *Designer polymeal*, for more hints and tips on optimal healthy eating.

Try another idea...

Now, your homocysteine level is naturally determined by your genes. But taking folic acid at doses of 0.5–5.0 mg a day has been found to lower raised homocysteine concentrations by about 25%. Taking 0.5 mg per day of vitamin B12, too, reduces raised homocysteine levels by a further 7%. This amount of reduction of homocysteine in the bloodstream has been calculated to reduce the risks of a further heart attack or stroke in someone who already has coronary heart disease – by as much as 30%. The American Heart Association (www.americanheart.org), and other similar national organisations elsewhere, do not recommend the use of folic acid and vitamin B supplements to reduce the risks of heart disease or stroke, however. Instead they advise you to get them through a healthy balanced diet that includes at least five servings of fruit or leafy green vegetables a day. Aim for a daily intake of 400 micrograms of folic acid or folate: citrus fruits, tomatoes, vegetables and grain products are good sources.

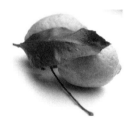

'Knowledge is power.'
SIR FRANCIS BACON, British adventurer, politician and writer

Defining idea...

How did it go?

Q **My parents both died from heart disease in their forties and I don't want to go the same way. I don't smoke, I take lots of exercise and I try to keep my weight down. Should I have my homocysteine levels checked?**

A *At present there's generally thought to be insufficient evidence to warrant routine measurement of homocysteine levels in the bloodstream, but this may change in the future as more research is published. However, people like you – people who don't have any risk factors other than a strong family history of heart disease – might benefit from homocysteine screening and treatment with folic acid supplements if their homocysteine levels are found to be high. It is getting much easier to check homocysteine levels, so ask your doctor's advice and see if they are prepared to check it for you.*

Q **Can I control my homocysteine levels through what I eat?**

A *Well, eating lots of fruit and vegetables reduces the likelihood of someone developing heart disease, and this happens to be the best sort of diet for boosting your folic acid intake, too. So eat plenty of fruit and nuts, breakfast cereals, lentils, green leafy veg such as spinach – and root vegetables, beans and mushrooms. Don't be too liberal with the amount of animal protein you eat, avoid refined carbohydrates and only drink alcohol in moderation. That's the best you can do to help yourself. But there is definitely a school of thought that advocates taking a multivitamin containing folate and the B vitamins – and as it won't do you any harm, why not do that too?*

14

Salt away

When is it good to be down and out? When it's salt you're talking about – cut it down or cut it out...

Too much salt can lead to high blood pressure — increasing your risk of heart disease. So the less salt you have, the better.

Reducing salt works. Having more salt in your diet triggers heart disease and raised blood pressure. We don't know why, but too much salt can give you acid reflux, too.

Most people consume around 10 g of salt a day – but if you like salty food, you could be eating twice as much. Try to have less than 6 g of salt in total per day: that's about one level teaspoon. You probably don't have much of a clue about how much salt is in the food you eat – how much is in your basic food, not just what you add to your cooking or sprinkle on afterwards, and it can be fiddly to find out. Processed foods – such as canned soups, sausages, meat pies, take-aways and other ready prepared meals – are stuffed with salt. Bread, and some cereals, have salt added to heighten their taste, and these are foods you might not suspect of being high in salt. The ones which are typically full of salt are crisps, nuts, pork pies and pizzas.

Salt is often given as sodium on food labels. This isn't very helpful, but 2.5 g of sodium is equivalent to 6 g of salt, and 0.5 g or more of sodium per 100 g of food is

Here's an idea for you... **Get hold of a salt calculator to help encourage you to cut your salt intake. The credit-card-sized calculator can help you to measure your salt consumption and convert sodium to salt quantities. If you can't find one in the shops, they're available online.**

an awful lot of salt; less than 0.1 g of sodium per 100 g of food is a little salt. If you go and look at a tin of baked beans, you'll probably find it contains about 1 g of sodium per serving, and remember to take the size of helping into account and not just the concentration of salt. Foods like marmite have a high salt content, but you only use a little bit, whereas a helping of baked beans is two-fifths of the maximum salt intake you should have in an entire day.

Here's some advice on cutting down.

First, cut out or reduce the 25% or so of your daily salt intake that comes from adding salt to food while you're cooking or eating. If you can't, consider switching to a low-salt alternative: these contain up to two-thirds less sodium by substituting potassium chloride – unless there's a reason you should avoid extra potassium in your diet. You can cut down gradually; you're trying to reverse the bad habits of a lifetime, after all. Leave out foods that are high in salt and move to ones that are healthier. This might involve a complete rethink of your diet or a simple change to alternative cereals or breads, for example. Avoid salty snacks, choosing a piece of fruit or carrot instead (you angel, you!) and buy canned food that states 'no added salt'. Make your own sauces from scratch rather than buying prepared ones which are high in salt. Shake the salt cellar once instead of twice or more. As you get used to less salt you might actually find that your food is tastier: too much salt can mask the flavour.

Secondly, remember that what you see is what you get. Packaged food has nutritional information on the labels, so read them before you put your shopping in your trolley. Look at the amount per serving for pre-prepared food, and not just at the amount per 100 g which will probably be much less (and bear in mind that some manufacturers' ideas of what a 'serving' is may not be the same as yours). For crisps and nuts look at the amount per packet; assume you'll eat the lot...

Check out IDEA 15, *Get it down*, for some more motivation on just why you should cut your salt levels.

Try another idea...

There are lots of myths around salt. Don't believe things like these:

- 'Posh salt is better for you than table salt.' No, it isn't! It doesn't matter how much the salt costs or where it comes from. It's the sodium it contains that does the damage.
- 'You need to use more salt when it's hot or when you get overheated from playing sports because you sweat it out.' Not true. You lose a small amount of salt in sweat and that's easily covered by your everyday food.

And there are lots more where those came from. Don't fall for them.

'Good habits result from resisting temptation.'
Ancient proverb

Defining idea...

Q **I have sprinkled salt over my food for the last thirty years. How can I break my bad habit?**

A *Try adding mixed herbs, garlic or ginger while cooking to give your food more flavour. That way you won't need to sprinkle salt on at the table or even in cooking. Your taste buds will adapt to the change pretty quickly and soon you won't miss it. Put your salt at the back of a cupboard and only bring it out for guests. And don't put those little salt packets on your tray in canteens or cafés – once you're at the table it will be too much bother to go back to collect the salt and you'll do without. Promise!*

Q **Is sea salt lower in sodium than common salt?**

A *No. Sea salt is sodium chloride too, but extracted from the sea rather than from the ground.*

Q **What kind of low-salt ready meals can I eat that are easy to cook up when I'm home late?**

A *Anything, provided you don't buy them; make up your own and you'll know what's gone into them. Use lemon, limes and oranges to flavour meat dishes. Make a stash of salt-free stock from stewing vegetables and use it for making sauces and gravy for your main meals and casseroles. Freeze tubs of that too.*

15

Get it down

How do you measure up? A bit like a tarot reading, your blood pressure levels predict your health in the future, but they're much more likely to come true.

The higher your blood pressure, the shorter your life expectancy, but the only way you'll know if you've got high blood pressure is to have it measured.

One in four of us has high blood pressure. Just bringing high blood pressure down by around 5% reduces your risk of having a heart attack or angina by a fifth.

The medical term for blood pressure that remains high is hypertension. Blood pressure is the force with which blood is pumped around the body. When it's high, the heart has to work much harder to keep the circulation going. It changes depending on what you're doing; when you're asleep it falls and when you're having sex it rises (the blood pressure, that is).

There's nothing good about high blood pressure – except for the drug firms who make healthy profits from people on their treatments. Mind you, they do miss out on some fat profits as a third of people with high blood pressure don't know they've got it. If your blood pressure's been high for a long time your heart will grow larger to stand up to the extra pressures on it, and will be less efficient.

Here's an idea for you... **Buy a home monitor to take your own blood pressure at the touch of a button. Go for a digital electronic one that has been validated by the professionals (check that out at www.dableducational.org) and don't buy a wrist or finger monitoring device. Make sure the cuff is the right size for your arm. It's not that you can do better than the professionals, it's just that you'll be more relaxed at home and they'll be more likely to be true readings. Keep records of your blood pressure at different times of day – expect it to be lower at night than in the morning and to shoot up a bit if you're under stress. Don't get obsessed, though. Check it every month or so unless there's a reason to do it more often. And ask your doctor for a personal plan so you can adjust your own blood pressure drugs**

The next thing you know, you could develop heart failure – making it even more likely that you'll have a heart attack.

If you've currently got a reckless lifestyle, then make a change. Go for a low-fat, high-fibre diet, increase the amount of fruit and veg you eat, cut the salt, eat oily fish, lose weight, take regular dynamic exercise, limit the amount of alcohol you drink, stop smoking, reduce your stress… You've heard all that before – but you might not be doing as much as you can, though. If you're obese, even a 10% weight loss can bring your high blood pressure down to normal levels. And increasing the amount of fibre in your diet can drive your blood pressure down too.

There are more than a hundred drugs to control high blood pressure. On the whole, it's better to have lower amounts of two or more drugs combined, than too much of one drug. They have names that make no sense but sound impressive: ACE inhibitors, angiotensin-II antagonists, thiazide diuretics, beta-blockers and calcium channel blockers. As there's not much difference in power between these drugs, doctors tend to prescribe the least expensive ones. Some are better than others for elderly people with high blood pressure, some are better for certain ethnic groups, or for people who've got diabetes too. Combining three drugs that lower blood pressure can cut your chances of having a heart attack by half.

Another good thing about there being so many drugs for blood pressure – except for keeping drug manufacturers' families clothed and fed – is that you can swop the various drugs if you do get side effects like tiredness, swollen ankles, cold hands and feet (and impotence in men). If you overdo the drugs and your blood pressure plummets too low you might feel dizzy or faint. One other thing: leave off any herbal or homeopathic remedies you've bought yourself until you're sure they don't clash with any medication you've been prescribed by your doctor or nurse.

As well as taking drugs to lower your high blood pressure, you may be best taking a low dose of aspirin, see IDEA 17, *Aspirin – the truth.*

Try another idea...

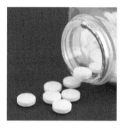

'What goes up must come down.'
British proverb

Defining idea...

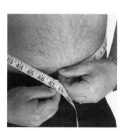

How did it go?

Q   My mum often gets nosebleeds but won't go to the doctor as she says it's nothing. Do you think she could have high blood pressure?

A   *Nosebleeds can sometimes be a sign of high blood pressure, but for most people there'll be other reasons. She won't know unless she gets her blood pressure checked. She could go to a doctor or nurse at her local clinic or, if she doesn't want to do that, maybe a pharmacist could take it.*

Q   Should a man have the same blood pressure as a woman?

A   *Yes, in this area men and women are just the same. Blood pressure is measured in millimetres of mercury (written as mmHg) and written up as a fraction, with one figure on top of the other. Normal pressures are a maximum of 160/90 (160 systolic and 90 diastolic), but if you've already got heart disease you'll want your blood pressure to be below 140/85. It's even more critical to get it as low as 130/80 if you've got diabetes too.*

Q   I keep fit and eat well. Why have I got high blood pressure?

A   *There's often no obvious cause. If your parents had high blood pressure, then you're more likely to have it too. Otherwise, being overweight, using too much salt or drinking too much alcohol could be putting your pressure up. Just make sure you've not got kidney disease – that's a rare cause – and check it's not a side effect of any drug you're on. Your blood pressure will rise a bit as you get older, too.*

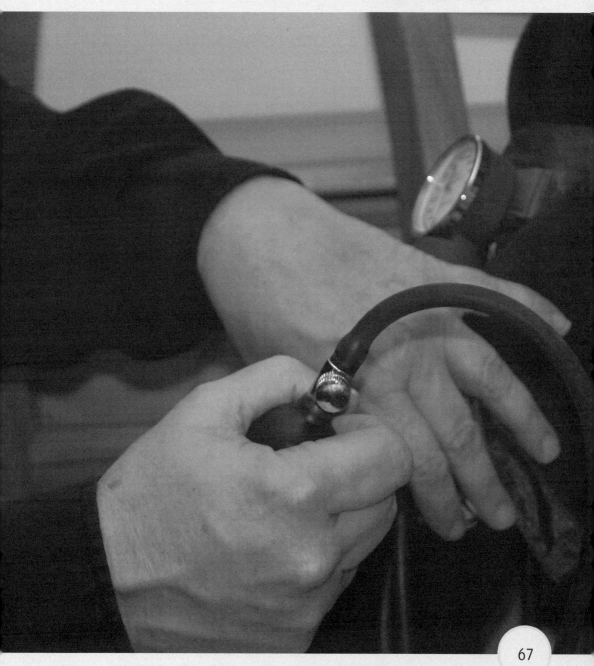

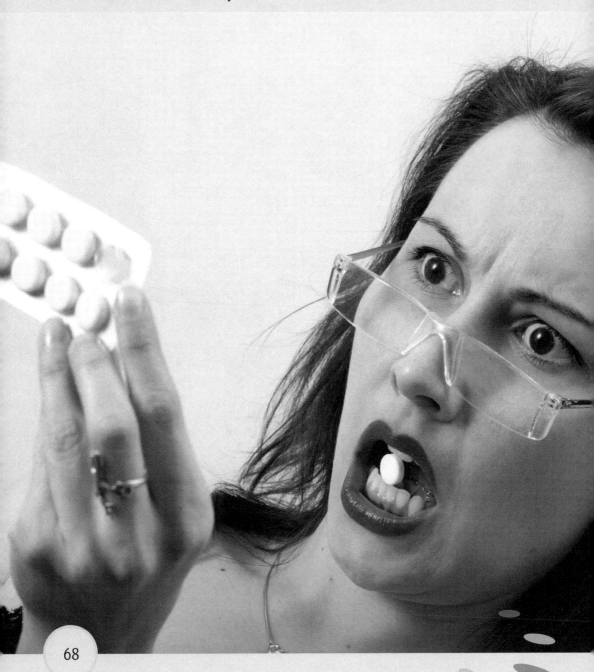

16

Take that

Trust them, they're doctors, nurses, pharmacists, even advertising executives. They know what drugs are good for you and your heart, or your blood pressure (well, maybe not the advertising executives).

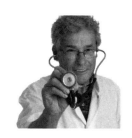

Primary prevention means your doctor or nurse prescribing drugs for you if you're at risk of a heart attack. Secondary prevention uses similar drugs — to stop people with heart troubles getting any worse or having a repeat attack. So what should you take?

The 'should I, shouldn't I, take it' debate is often about who should take statins and when, and for what level of cholesterol. Then there's the debate about what kind of drug to take to thin your blood and stop it clotting if you're at risk, such as from heart valve disease or after a stroke. Controversy over drugs that lower blood pressure surrounds how a person's blood pressure level is established. Should you take any drugs if your blood pressure is only raised when being checked by the doctor, if it's pretty normal the rest of the time?

Here's an idea for you...

About half the medicines prescribed for people with chronic health problems are not taken. Concordance means that you, the patient, take an equal part with the medic advising you in making a decision about what treatment you'll take. Don't rely only on the internet for information; much of it's too general, incomplete, irrelevant or wrong. Find medical advisers you trust and get them to give you high-quality information. Reflect on it, formulate questions and get answers. Then you're ready to make big decisions with your doctor about the treatment options – and the risks and benefits for you.

If you look round the internet for guidance on preventing or treating heart disease, you'll see lots of different advice given in lots of different countries, even on official websites. Health service management people take into account the stupendous cost of supplying drugs to their population depending on the thresholds set for treatment, and any deals they can negotiate with pharmaceutical companies. Economists consider whether it's worth treating people with high cholesterol if they've no other risks of heart disease, such as diabetes or smoking. Will the payback be worth the investment in drugs if someone has got at least a one in three, or a one in ten, chance of dying in the next ten years? Faceless committees make these decisions and then the communications specialists spring into action to convey their guidance as fact. And it's very easy to be swayed by marketing ads targeted directly at you – personalised for your age, gender and circumstances, so as to engage your interest and, often, your wallet. Don't make any decisions without seeing a doctor or healthcare professional and discussing them fully.

There are other things to consider, too. Tablets you take for one condition can react with other drugs, including some that are available without prescription. So declare everything else you're taking when seeing your doctor, and always check with the instructions in the packets when you're buying remedies yourself. See if there could be clashes with what you're already taking.

If you've had any recent heart problems, then taking drugs like Viagra could make things worse. Check out IDEA 46, *Early to bed*.

Try another idea...

Now, sometimes your risk of a heart attack can soar when you stop taking certain drugs. That's not just the preventive kind, like statins and aspirin, but also ones such as anti-inflammatory drugs for joint pains. If you're curious, you can scour medical journals yourself to look at your increased risks of having a heart attack or stroke while you're taking anti-inflammatory drugs, for example, though medics are still confused as to the extent to which some drugs increase your risks while others lower them – check out www.annals.org. It's not just joint drugs that can cause heart attacks, but antipsychotic drugs too, for instance. They probably give the user three times the risk of sudden death – not that you'd be weighing the risk like this if you were in such a bad state as to need to take that kind of heavy drug.

'When we want your opinion, we'll give it to you.'
Caption to a cartoon in a medical journal

Defining idea...

How did it go?

Q My sister and I recently shared a bedroom when we went away together. When we compared our tablets, we found we were taking exactly the same ones. We were flabbergasted, as mine are because my blood pressure is high and my sister has never had problems with her blood pressure at all. Is it safe to continue my treatment?

A *Many of the tablets for treating high blood pressure can be used for other conditions, so don't worry if your sister's taking the same drug as you, but for a different reason. It's really important to take your treatment regularly to keep your blood pressure down. Ask for more information about how your drugs work next time you go for a check up or collect them from the pharmacy.*

Q I've been on statins to lower my cholesterol level for several years. Every so often the nurse does a blood test to check my liver function, which seems to be up the creek, but they still tell me to keep taking the tablets. What do you think, are the statin drugs harming me?

A *Your physician will be watching the overactivity of your liver enzymes. So long as they're not more than three times the upper limit of normal, they'll advise you to continue with your statins as it's so important to keep your cholesterol level down. It's not your hectic social life and plenty of alcohol that's affecting your liver though, is it? If so, they'll want to review whether you should carry on taking those statins or not.*

17

Aspirin – the truth

Aspirin's a life-saver. And not just for relieving a throbbing headache, but for keeping you alive and well as long as possible.

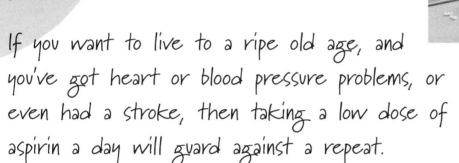

If you want to live to a ripe old age, and you've got heart or blood pressure problems, or even had a stroke, then taking a low dose of aspirin a day will guard against a repeat.

The evidence is pretty clear-cut. There are no overall health benefits from taking a regular aspirin for those people who have a healthy heart, as far as they know, and a normal blood pressure. So even if you've got close relatives who have dropped dead at an early age of a heart attack, or who have had high blood pressure or heart failure, there's no point taking aspirin to try and prevent yourself going the same way. The best you can do is to continue with your healthy lifestyle and happy life. Don't take an aspirin a day 'just in case', either, as aspirin can cause bleeding in the stomach for people who are susceptible, which is risky in itself.

But if you're someone who's got heart or blood pressure problems or who's had a stroke, the picture's completely different. You must take a low dose of aspirin a day

Here's an idea for you... **Take a one-off low dose of aspirin before you travel a long distance by car or plane. Go for a 75–150 mg dose a couple of hours before you leave to minimise the chance of a blood clot forming while you're sitting around. You can do leg exercises and deep breathing, too, to promote your circulation. They say that blood clots may form in the deep veins of as many as one in ten long-haul airline passengers, without them having had any symptoms and realising it. You're more at risk of getting one of these deep vein thromboses if you're obese, aged over forty, already have heart problems, are pregnant, on the oral contraceptive pill or hormone replacement therapy (HRT), or even if you're dehydrated, maybe from drinking too much alcohol or from severe diarrhoea.**

– 75 mg will do. If you know you've got any kind of diabetes, you're also in the group who'll benefit from taking an aspirin a day. It'll bring down the odds of you having a heart attack or stroke by 20–30% and that level of improvement in your chances has got to be worth having. If you've got angina, then taking a low dose of aspirin every day will reduce your chances of a heart attack, and of actually dying from a heart attack, by at least 50% – and aspirin is given after heart bypass surgery, too. In fact, aspirin's so powerful that 150–300 mg of aspirin is one of the emergency treatments that doctors and paramedics give immediately, when they see someone with chest pain and suspect they're having a heart attack or stroke (the emergency dose is much bigger than the everyday, slow dose). The soluble kind acts most quickly.

Now, the higher the dose of aspirin you take, the more chance it will give you a bleed – from your stomach or brain or elsewhere in your body. So it's safer to take 75 mg of aspirin, or acetylsalicyclic acid, every day than the 150 or even 300 mg a day that some experts recommend. And it looks as if the benefits of

taking 300 mg of aspirin a day are pretty much
the same as those from taking 75 mg, though
some doctors think that people with diabetes
might be better on the higher dose. Some
individuals do develop a resistance to aspirin
when they've been on it for a long time, and sometimes other alternative drugs are
added or substituted to stop a blood clot forming. Research that followed
thousands of middle-aged men for up to four years showed that for every thousand
taking a low dose of aspirin, fifty-five did not have a heart attack or stroke or fatal
episode that they could otherwise have been expected to have; eight bled from
their guts because they'd taken it, however. If you've had a bleeding duodenal ulcer
in the past, you wouldn't want to risk that happening again; after all, there are
other drugs that can make your blood less sticky if you can't take aspirin.

**Check out IDEA 16, *Take that,*
to understand more about the
drugs you take.**

*Try
another
idea...*

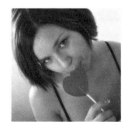 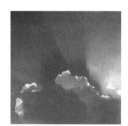

*'The people that walked in
darkness have seen a great
light: they that dwell in the
land of the shadow of death,
upon them hath the light
shined.'*
The Bible

*Defining
idea...*

75

How did it go?

Q **Is there any way to minimise the chances that I will suffer harm from taking aspirin?**

A *Aspirin will be less likely to irritate your stomach if you take it after food. You can also get enteric-coated aspirin; that has a slower action as it isn't absorbed as quickly as ordinary aspirin preparations. That slow action will suit you, though, if you're taking it to prevent yourself from having a heart attack or stroke, when you want a low dose to be trickling steadily through your bloodstream.*

Q **My stomach is like iron, so I don't think I'll have any trouble with aspirin. Are there any other side effects that I should be worried about?**

A *Well, it's not a good idea to make assumptions here. Even if you can eat an extra-hot curry without suffering for it, you can't be sure that aspirin won't cause bleeding if you're susceptible; it's not the same. If you're on other drugs, such as anti-inflammatory drugs or antidepressants, check with your doctor that aspirin is safe for you to take regularly. It can increase your risk of bleeding when combined with these and loads of other drugs.*

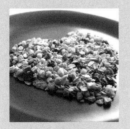 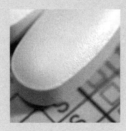

18

Loads of alternatives

Do you use complementary medicine? Once people might have thought you were weird, but these days so many of us use complementary medicines, you'd be weird not to give one a try.

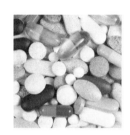

Many complementary and alternative medicines are based on the opinion that they probably work, rather than lots of evidence that they actually cure people. But there's little evidence that they don't work, either.

Some complementary practitioners are also doctors, physiotherapists or nurses who are state registered with their own professional bodies. Others, such as osteopaths and chiropractors, are registered with their own statutory bodies; in France and Germany, it's mostly medically trained doctors who practise complementary therapy. Most complementary practitioners have completed some form of further education in their discipline. But their knowledge and skills mainly come from training based on what has been passed down by tradition rather than actually proven by hard scientific evidence. That's no reason to write them off, however.

Here's an idea for you... **Many of the alternative therapies involve other people touching you with their hands. The exclusive attention of a therapist in treating you for fifteen minutes or more can make you feel good and cared for; you'll leave an alternative therapy session feeling marvellous after this kind of treatment. With conventional health care, a prescription for a drug promises benefits sometime in the future, not right now, in the present. Maybe you could pick and mix complementary therapies and conventional health care with the same practitioner – they can coexist and you'll be the winner. Don't go to more than one practitioner at a time, though; their treatments might conflict and they won't necessarily know what each other is doing.**

There are physical, psychological, social and spiritual problems connected to all human illness. Your body has the capacity for self-repair. A complementary practitioner treats each person as an individual. Their holistic package of care for you will include advice about your lifestyle, counselling, relaxation, diet and exercise as well as their particular therapy for your troubles and symptoms.

There are some common features between the various kinds of complementary therapies. Some of the terms used such as 'oi/chi' or 'prana energy' have no equivalent in Western medical culture. Such energy is thought to travel through channels – chakras or meridians – as in acupuncture. Diseases of specific organs or systems of the body are linked to particular mental or emotional patterns of symptoms; for example, anxiety and fear might cause digestive disturbances: you'll know that from when you get a dodgy stomach on the morning of an exam or before an important interview. Holistic treatments try to clear and balance these disturbed energies by working on your body's self-healing capacity and provoking a positive immune response rather than targeting specific symptoms or diseases. Many doctors and nurses practise in this holistic manner too. Holistic practitioners believe that your illness provides you with an opportunity for making positive changes as you create a better balance to your life.

Check out IDEA 51, *Relaxing you*, to read about more ways of using complementary therapies.

Try another idea...

Some people try complementary medicine because they're desperate, when they've tried all the conventional treatments without success. Others like alternative medicines because they seem low-tech compared to conventional healthcare, or may be sceptical about the benefits or dangers of conventional treatments prescribed by doctors. The feeling of being in control of the various treatments – because you pay for complementary therapies – appeals to some people. There are so many different approaches that you should find something to help you: so long as you can afford it.

On the whole, we don't know how many of the alternative therapies are effective for exactly which conditions; for example, just because acupuncture is effective for lower back pain, doesn't necessarily mean that it's also effective for controlling or preventing chest pain or angina. Most people don't care why a certain remedy works, just that it does. And for some it might be the placebo effect – the fact that they're taking a treatment – that makes them think it's working. If someone listens to you with interest and uses their hands to massage or treat you, you're likely to leave them feeling better. And the jury is still out in many areas: lots of people advocate various vitamins for preventing heart disease, for instance, while others report that multivitamins cannot stop people with heart problems having further heart attacks or strokes.

'Let's be clear about the boundaries. A broken leg requires hospitalisation, full stop. A diseased appendix needs to be removed, full stop. But recovery from appendicitis is likely to be aided by complementary care and a strong immune system.'
PETER HAIN, UK politician

Defining idea...

How did it go?

Q I'm confused, as there are so many alternatives to choose from with lots of pros and cons. How can I be sure what treatment I'm getting and what it will do?

A   *Be ready with a checklist of questions and go through them with the therapist when you're considering trying any new treatment. These are the sort of things you could ask: What will this treatment do? How long will I need to be treated for? How much will it cost? Can I take this treatment alongside other treatments or medicines I'm taking? What are my chances of side effects or after effects? This should help clear up your confusion.*

Q Complementary treatments sound safer than conventional medicines. Are they?

A   *Well, not enough is known about which complementary and alternative medicines do more good than harm. Some forms are safe, but others aren't, so be cautious and do some research yourself. Be careful that you don't get side effects from a clash between therapies, such as a medication prescribed by a doctor and herbal medicine bought over the counter. Always tell your doctor or pharmacist what complementary treatments you're taking, or check carefully on the packet of any complementary therapies you're buying if you're already on prescribed drugs.*

19

Herbs-enlist

Plant an idea in your head about the great effects of some herbal medicines...

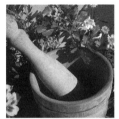

Herbal medicine makes use of the healing properties of plants and herbs. They've been used to treat illness and injury for thousands of years.

They're made from roots, flowers, herbs, bark or plant extracts, and the herbalist may use the whole plant to make up the remedy. They're one of the most popular forms of complementary medicine – 10% of adults in the US take herbal medicines.

Herbal medicines might help if you're suffering from heart failure or a high cholesterol level. After all, digoxin is the mainstream treatment throughout the world for helping failing hearts to beat strongly, and was originally derived from foxgloves in the eighteenth century. Herbal medicines today are usually used for generalised conditions, acting through their anti-inflammatory or antispasmodic properties. The top ten herbs bought in the US include five taken for heart-related reasons – garlic, kava kava, ginkgo biloba, ginseng and St John's Wort.

Here's an idea for you... **You deserve a specialised consultation with an experienced herbalist; don't just try off-the-shelf herbal medicine in a happy-go-lucky way. Then you'll get a specific herbal remedy tailored to your current symptoms, general health and lifestyle, previous and other illnesses. So look in the phone book, or ask friends for recommendations and make a date with a qualified herbalist.**

- Garlic is used as a food and herb in many countries and has been used in most cultures for preventing and treating infections and maintaining general health. It is frequently used to prevent arteriosclerosis and lower cholesterol. Take 4 g of fresh garlic or 8 mg of garlic oil, or 600–900 mg of standardised extract a day.

- Kava kava is used more for treating anxiety and difficulties in sleeping which helps your heart indirectly. Go for 300 mg of standardised extract over your day.

- Ginkgo biloba is a top-selling herbal remedy for high blood pressure and angina, among other things. 120–160 mg of standardised extract over a day helps with circulation problems, so you can walk further without getting pain in your legs.

- Ginseng is sometimes used for heart failure, but it's not as effective as prescribed medication from a doctor; its adverse effects probably outweigh its benefits. It's used to promote health and longevity and aid convalescence.

- St John's Wort is an extract from the hypericum bush. Doses vary from 300–1000 mg a day. This is more for any underlying anxiety and depression you've got, rather than for having a direct effect on your heart. Side effects may include oversensitivity to light, the formation of cataracts in the eyes, stomach upsets, tiredness and restlessness. St John's Wort can also interact with things such as contraceptives, blood-thinning tablets, heart tablets, antidepressant drugs and epileptic treatments – so take care and check with your doctor first before taking it.

Most herbal remedies prescribed by a qualified and experienced herbalist are safe. But just because herbal medicines are 'natural' doesn't mean that they're guaranteed to be safe and some are highly toxic. Sometimes, conventional medication has been added to what looks like herbal medicine in order to increase its effectiveness. If your herbal remedy already contains paracetamol, diazepam or even steroids, you can see how easily you might overdose if you're already on similar medication.

Herbal cigarettes might see you through while you're getting over your addiction to standard ones, though they're heavy on tar and carbon monoxide. For more ideas on stopping smoking, look at IDEA 39, *Quit!*

Try another idea...

Although rare, there are fatalities. Even warfarin, used to thin the blood, has been found in herbal medicine intended to treat prostate disease. Liquorice root can cause you to retain sodium in your body and push your blood pressure up. Yohimbe bark, used as an aphrodisiac or for impotence by some men, can cause the heart to beat very fast or irregularly. Ma Huang, an asthma remedy, can push your blood pressure up too and make your heart beat erratically and even lead to sudden death.

Chinese remedies for skin conditions commonly contain steroids. As well as lead,

'Better be safe than sorry.'
English proverb

Defining idea...

mercury and arsenic, some herbal medicines contain tin or silver – all of which can cause you serious harm. You can suffer adverse effects such as diarrhoea or anaemia or even the worsening of other diseases such as schizophrenia. In addition herbal remedies may interact with medication prescribed by a doctor or that you buy in a store. This can trigger side effects and might heighten the effect of the conventional drug you've been prescribed. For instance, if you suffer from epilepsy and took evening primrose oil alongside your anticonvulsant treatment, you'd be more likely to have fits, not less. And one final word: don't risk taking herbal medicines if you're pregnant unless advised by a doctor.

Q **Are herbal medicines regulated in any way?**

A *The source and quality of most herbal remedies aren't standardised and they're not subject to such strict controls as are regulated pharmaceutical medicines – yet.*

Q **How do I find a herbalist I can trust?**

A *There are various national bodies, depending on where you live. Do some research on the internet, make a few calls and check that your herbalist is a member of a professional association or linked to a national association or a similar body.*

Q **What precautions can I take to be sure that any herbal medicine I try is safe?**

A *Read the packet to check it's safe for you, or ask the pharmacist or health store adviser. Tell them about other medication you're taking so you avoid any interactions. When consulting a doctor or nurse, tell them what herbal medicines you're taking before they give you a prescription. Take the packet along so they can read up on the ingredients. You might have to be ready to stop your herbal remedy while you're taking a conventionally prescribed treatment.*

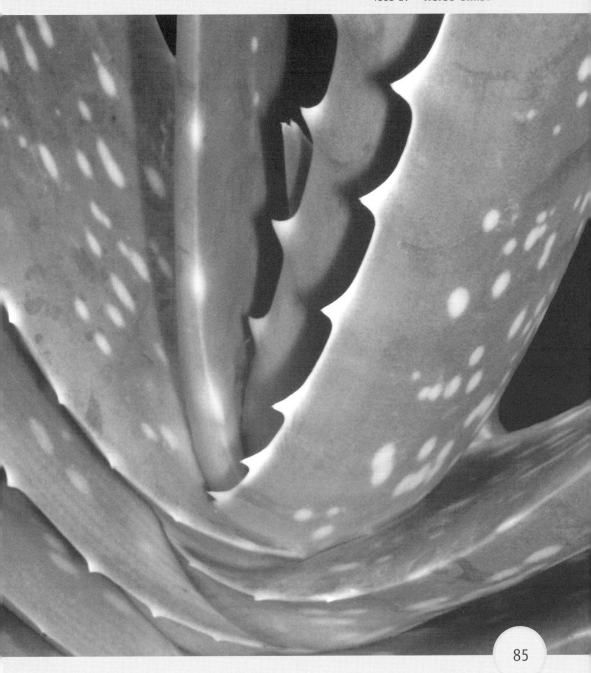

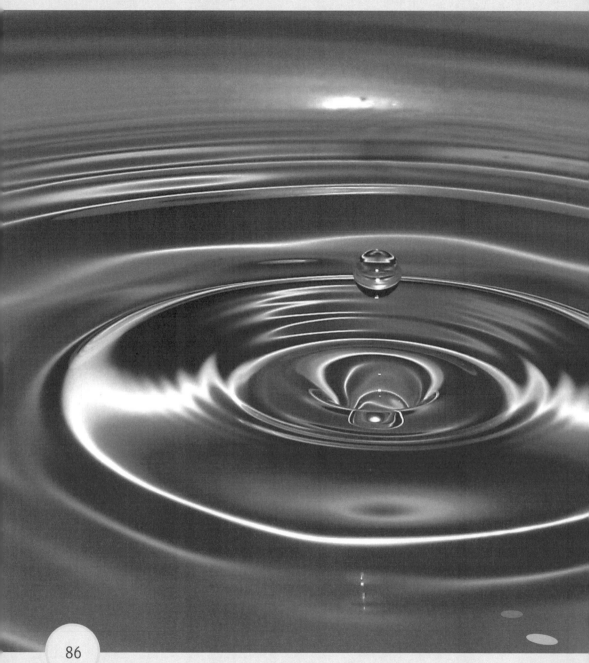

20

Hypnotherapy

Here's a puzzle for you. What's the link between hypnotherapy and hearts, apart from both words starting with the same letter? Well, hypnotherapy can help you be rid of the bad habits that threaten the health of your heart.

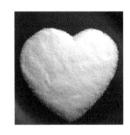

Hypnosis is used for all sorts of psychosomatic conditions: anxiety, stress, pain, addictions and phobia. So, to keep your heart healthy, that's help with stopping smoking, losing weight and relieving your stress if you're over-hyped.

With hypnosis you'll be in a trance-like state where you're so deeply relaxed that you'll be open to suggestions and suspend your critical faculties. Your conscious mind is subdued; your unconscious mind lies ready and waiting for those suggestions. The hypnotherapist will generally see you in their consulting room – somewhere quiet, fairly dark and private. You'll sit in a comfortable armchair where you can lean back and relax, with the hypnotherapist sitting nearby. They'll start off by talking to you about your problems and what other approaches you've tried. You'll soon feel safe, so as to be able to relax into that hypnotic state.

Here's an
idea for
you...

If you've had a few successful sessions with a hypnotist, you're probably ready to try self-hypnosis. A hypnotist might work with you and a group of others to teach this technique. You can be given a suggestion while you're under hypnosis that enables you to induce self-hypnosis after the treatment course has finished, and with regular practice you'll be able to use it at will. Your self-hypnotic state will probably last about twenty minutes at a time. Visual cues such as looking at a particular picture of a seashore or imagining such a picture can trigger your own hypnotic state. Some people prefer to play a relaxation tape as a way of hypnotising themselves.

A session typically lasts between thirty and ninety minutes. The first visit will take longer, so that the hypnotherapist can hear about your problem and you can get to know and trust them. Usually you'll have six to twelve weekly sessions. Once the therapist has induced your hypnotic trance, they'll make therapeutic suggestions to change your behaviour or relieve your symptoms. You'll be in a state between waking and sleeping; aware of everything going on around you, but at the same time completely detached from it. Don't worry: you can end the trance anytime you want to – you're not powerless.

There are different techniques for inducing a hypnotic trance. Here's one way. You'll imagine that you're drifting comfortably away, and be picturing yourself in a tranquil setting such as an idyllic countryside scene. Your eyelids may feel heavy and your eyes will gradually close. Then the hypnotherapist will lead you to shift your attention from your external environment towards an object relating to your problem. The sort of suggestions they'll make will be for you to control your heart rate by imagining you're slowing down the ticking of a clock. Or they may suggest that smoking cigarettes is no longer something you actually want to do, so that after your hypnosis session smoking no longer dominates your life. Although you're open to suggestion, the hypnotherapist won't be able to make you do something you don't want to. Afterwards, you may not remember what happened to you or what suggestions were planted. Let's take smoking as an example. Hypnotherapy may weaken your desire to smoke and strengthen your will to stop. It can help you really focus or concentrate on what you've got to do. You'll hear that smoking is a poison, that your body is entitled to protection from smoke and about the advantages of being a non-smoker. As many as one in three smokers can give up with hypnotherapy.

There's also a form of hypnosis you can use yourself. The technique of autogenic training draws heavily from hypnosis and yoga. Almost anyone can learn autogenic training by reading a self-help book, and it can be mastered in only a few weeks. With autogenic training you focus on experiencing physical sensations such as warmth and heaviness in different parts of your body. You'll develop a sequence of very specific auto-suggestive formulae that you repeat in a particular pattern with formulised resolutions that you repeat up to thirty times. You could try learning meditation and relaxation techniques, too, as alternative ways to induce a really deeply relaxed state.

Hypnotherapy should be good for helping you to sleep much better, but look at IDEA 26, *Sleep, glorious sleep*, for other ways.

Try another idea...

'To change your mind and to follow him who sets you right is to be nonetheless the free agent that you were before.'
MARCUS AURELIUS

Defining idea...

89

How did
it go?

Q How do I find a hypnotherapist I can trust?

A You really do need to find someone trustworthy, because you'll be in a very vulnerable position when in a hypnotic trance. You want to be sure that your hypnotist is planting positive and helpful suggestions in your mind, rather than negative or playful ones. Some doctors, dentists or psychologists are trained in hypnotherapy and some provide hypnotherapy alongside conventional treatments. There are lots of non-medically qualified hypnotherapists too. There are various national bodies; check out the internet to find one for where you live. They'll have lists of registered practitioners.

Q I've tried hypnosis once before but had difficulty relaxing into a hypnotic state. Any tips?

A Imagine yourself in a tranquil setting. Practise before you go and think of a particular setting you'll be able to recall easily when you're at the hypnotism session. You could try holding a coin in your hand. Concentrate on that whilst you're talked into the hypnotic state. When the coin drops from your hand your eyes will close and your body relax fully.

Q I want to try hypnosis, but I've had a chequered life and I don't want hypnosis to dredge up my past. What should I do?

A Well, hypnosis can sometimes reawaken memories of something traumatic that you'd rather stayed buried. If you're upset or have mental health problems, then you're better avoiding it.

21

Not a little

If a little of what you fancy does you good, leave it at that – homeopathic heart helpers.

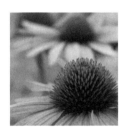

If a homeopathic remedy works, why risk the size effects of conventional medicine, thousands of times stronger?

The principle of homeopathy is that like cures like. A little of what makes you worse can also make you better. Substances that in large doses will cause the symptoms of an illness can be used in minute quantities to relieve the same symptoms.

Homeopathic remedies are derived from natural sources such as a mineral, a plant or an animal secretion. Plants used include the dangerous-sounding belladonna, arnica and chamomile. Minerals are those such as mercury and sulphur, and animal products include squid ink and snake venom. The remedies are prepared by repeated dilution and violent shaking. The more times this is repeated, the more potent the homeopathic remedy will be, and as a result there's very little active ingredient present. Because of this some people question whether homeopathic remedies can have any benefit at all, other than a placebo effect: working because you're told it will work, so it makes you feel better when you take it. Others believe that even very dilute homeopathic medicines act on people's biological function at the cellular level.

The idea is that homeopathy works by stimulating your body's capability to heal itself. So homeopathic medicine can only cure your health problems when your

Here's an idea for you...

Find a doctor who is also a homeopath, if you've got a heart condition and daren't try homeopathic treatment in case it clashes with the conventional drugs you're already taking. Then you won't worry if you get a brief aggravation of your symptoms. That's common when you start a homeopathic remedy – after all, that's how homeopathic medicine basically works.

body is actually able to repair itself; for more serious conditions, like heart failure, expect homeopathic remedies to lessen rather than actually cure your symptoms. You can buy homeopathic treatments from shops and pharmacies, or have them prescribed by homeopathic practitioners. Some are branded medicines and others are flower remedies. Some are single remedies, and others are combinations of three or four different ones. The drawback of off-the-shelf homeopathic medicines is that these are not specifically tailored to you, so your choice will be a bit hit and miss.

Homeopathic medicines with a wide spectrum of activity are called 'polychrests', while 'complex' remedies are a mixture of medicines, usually with specific uses. Homeopathic remedies may be given as tablets, granules, powders or in liquid form. They're usually dissolved in your mouth rather than swallowed and you shouldn't take food or drink for fifteen minutes or so before or after taking a remedy. The numbers after the names indicate the extent of dilution; '6c' is generally recommended for ailments which have developed over a longer period of time, whereas the stronger '30c' is generally used for acute conditions. Potentially toxic concentrations of some homeopathic drugs have been described, as have occasional allergic reactions.

There are more than 2000 substances used by homeopaths to treat diseases. Homeopathic medicines can help coughs and colds, digestive complaints, skin conditions and joint pains. And many homeopathic medicines are recommended for the heart and circulatory system.

Have a look at IDEA 18, *Loads of alternatives*, to learn more about complementary medicine.

Try another idea...

Let's look at some specific examples. Aconite, cactus, lilium tig, spongia, tabacum and other homeopathic remedies are recommended for the various pains of angina and accompanying symptoms, taken when symptoms occur and at intervals thereafter. Aurum met, baryta carb and lachesis are examples of remedies used twice daily in order to combat raised blood pressure. Remedies like coffea or aconite, aethusa or phosphorus, are reckoned to be good for palpitations – taken every twenty minutes until the palpitations have improved. Aconite, tabacum, morphinium and abies nig, among others, are remedies that can combat heartbeats that are too fast or too slow.

A homeopathic practitioner will specify which remedy is appropriate for your particular symptoms, and prescribe treatment until improvement occurs. You'll have a different remedy to someone else with the same condition, because it's matched to you, personally. For a chronic problem, the homeopath will expect you to take the remedy for some months. Side effects can occur and are more likely with the more concentrated doses. Your initial session may last more than an hour, as your practitioner will take a really detailed history from you, considering all your personality traits and habits as well as your symptoms. Your progress will be reviewed periodically and the nature or strength of the remedy will be adjusted as necessary. It'll be reduced as soon as your symptoms improve, and stopped if your symptoms seem to have been aggravated or if you're getting better.

'Every little helps.'
British proverb

Defining idea...

How did it go?

Q   How can I find a good, trustworthy homeopath?

A   Training in homeopathy can vary from forty hours for someone who's a doctor already, to a three-year university degree. Some doctors practise homeopathic medicine alongside conventional health care. There'll be different regulations depending on whatever country you live in, but there will also be a national association of some kind who will be able to help you. Time to do a bit of research...

Q   I've got a sensitive stomach. Are there any adverse effects from using homeopathic medicines I should be aware of?

A   Because homeopathic remedies are so dilute they are non-toxic and can be taken at all ages and during pregnancy. Most side effects of homeopathic medicines are mild and pass quickly. You could experience headaches, tiredness, skin rash, dizziness or diarrhoea, but stick with it as these type of symptoms will soon pass. Don't delay seeking medical help for something more serious, or that you find particularly worrying.

Q   I take homeopathic medicine, so is it OK to take other drugs prescribed by my doctor too?

A   Some homeopathic remedies can clash with conventional drugs. So check first with your doctor or tell your homeopathic practitioner what other medicines you're taking. Some drugs, like antibiotics and steroids, can block the actions of homeopathic drugs and render them useless.

22

Ban illicit drugs...

They don't just blow your mind; all of the illicit drugs can affect your heart too. If you're going to pot, then you need to become an ex-user.

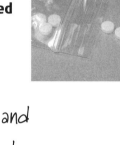

Some people try a drug like cannabis once, wonder what all the fuss is about and move on, but others really get hooked and develop extreme drug-related problems, including damaging effects on their health.

Let's look at different drugs and the effects they can have.

- If you smoke cannabis it will make your heart race, even at low doses. But, paradoxically, taking large doses will slow your heart rate down and lower your blood pressure. That leaves you four times more likely to have a heart attack in the hour after you've smoked cannabis. The effects of cannabis are directly proportional to how much you take, and a joint of the cannabis generally available today is many times stronger than it was when made up as a reefer twenty to thirty years ago. So you're more likely to suffer ill-effects now than you or your parents were in the '60s or '70s.

Here's an idea for you... **If you can't stop taking illicit drugs by yourself, get your family and friends to help you stop. Families Anonymous (www.famanon.org.uk) is a self-help, worldwide fellowship of families of drug users who share common problems. It helps and supports families, partners and friends. Now, it might be that your family may be inadvertently encouraging you to continue your drug habit by trying to protect you from the consequences of your addiction. See a drugs counsellor or specialist – what kind will depend on what kind of drugs you are addicted to and for how long you've had a problem.**

■ Cocaine constricts your blood vessels which gives you an unnatural high. Well, an unnaturally high blood pressure, too, soon after you've taken it. People mistakenly think that cocaine is a 'safer' option than many other drugs because it's traditionally snorted through straws or banknotes rather than being injected straight into a vein. But the constriction of the blood supply to your heart can give you chest pain – and, yes, even a heart attack. Compared to cannabis, you're much more likely to have a heart attack soon after using cocaine – twenty-three times more likely, in fact! Over time, the arteries in your heart can become badly furred up with persistent cocaine use, because of the massive rises and then sudden falls in blood pressure.

■ Ecstasy causes a fast heart rate and an associated rise in your blood pressure. People using ecstasy can die from it triggering funny heart rhythms or from having a stroke. If you don't actually die, you can be left paralysed by the stroke for the rest of your life...

■ Heroin is known to slow the breathing rate so much that you can actually stop breathing altogether and have a heart attack, or cardiac arrest. It slows your heart rate and lowers your blood pressure too. Injecting it can lead to the heart becoming infected when infection tracks round the blood system from a dirty injection site, or you can get a deep venous thrombosis or clot from injecting heroin in your groin.

You might have a problem with alcohol too, so try IDEA 23, *Booze over*, for help.

Try another idea...

■ Using glue and other solvents doesn't sound quite as serious as taking other illegal drugs, but they can trigger an abnormal heart rhythm which can be so hit and miss as to cause sudden death. The glue can affect the heart muscle itself resulting in a cardiomyopathy – chronic disease of the heart muscle.

Now you know – time to kick the habit. Let's take one example. In the case of cannabis, stopping smoking can help. Understand your use – do you crave a joint when you're stressed or nervous, after a meal, or when out with a particular group of friends? Avoid those situations where you know you'll be tempted and maybe unable to resist. Think of the effects your smoking has on your work, your family and friends, not just on your health. Once you've stopped, replace your habit with something new – a new hobby, new ways of spending your free time.

'Oh I get by with a little help from my friends,
Mm, I get high with a little help from my friends...'
JOHN LENNON and PAUL McCARTNEY – the song was originally written for Ringo Starr

Defining idea...

Q I thought cannabis had been used as a medicine for millions of years in China and the Middle East. So how can it really be dangerous?

A *Its reputation as a safe drug is unjustified. It's not lethal in the way that heroin is, but people often get addicted slowly and surely over time. It's not in the premier league of dangerous substances, but there are loads of health problems associated with it, not just the effects on your heart. You're more likely to get lung cancer from cannabis than ordinary tobacco and then there's anxiety and depression, psychotic states lasting for days, an increased risk of developing schizophrenia and more...*

Q Whatever, surely I'm better off taking cannabis and cocaine... they relax me and that's got to be good for my heart, hasn't it?

A *Drugs like cannabis and cocaine or alcohol are 'false friends' that give you the illusion of temporary relief from your stress and anxiety, but in reality they make it more difficult for you to sort out the problems that are causing you the stress in the first place. So trust me, I'm a doctor, your heart really will benefit if you stop using.*

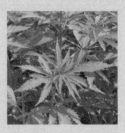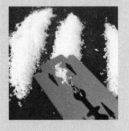

23

Booze over

Are you dying for a drink? Call a halt on your drinking if you're overdoing it – you might be surprised at how little is 'too much'.

It's a sobering thought, but as many as one in five people are drinking an unhealthy amount of alcohol.

Drinking too much alcohol triggers high blood pressure and that in turn can harm your heart from the extra pressure, or make you more likely to have a stroke. Let's get into some details.

There's one unit of alcohol in half a pint of standard-strength beer or lager, a small glass of wine (125 ml) at 9% proof, or a measure (25 ml) of spirits or fortified wine (50 ml) such as sherry. Some authorities give top weekly limits of alcohol as being fourteen units for a woman and twenty-one units for a man. Others say daily limits are more important and that a woman should drink no more than two to three units a day, and men no more than three to four units a day – with one or two days in the week being completely alcohol free. Having a weekly limit might encourage you to binge and drink all your weekly allowance on one night – and such bingeing is really bad for your liver. Women are more sensitive to the adverse effects of

Here's an idea for you...

Ask for help. That's easier than it sounds. Most people who realise they're drinking too much alcohol hide it from their family, their work colleagues and their doctor to start with. Own up to it. Until you face up to the fact you've got a problem you won't beat it. Complete the CAGE quiz: Have you ever felt the need to Cut down your drinking? Have people ever Annoyed you by complaining about your drinking? Have you ever felt Guilty about your drinking? Have you ever had an Eye-opener: a drink first thing in the morning to ease a hangover? Two or more positive answers, and you've got a problem, so go to a doctor or an alcohol counsellor.

alcohol than men, partly because they're smaller and have a higher proportion of body fat than men do.

Tot up how many units of alcohol you're really drinking. Keep a daily chart for a month. And do be honest – if you're not you're only fooling yourself. Anything over the recommended limits is too much. If you're worried, you could always have a blood test of your liver and the size of your blood cells. These can be normal though, or abnormal for different reasons – nothing to do with the alcohol you're drinking. A doctor might spot other signs that your liver is being damaged by alcohol if they examine you, and if they do so would probably arrange an ultrasound test of your liver to look at its texture and shape.

Now, you may be wondering what this has to do with your heart. If you're especially sensitive to alcohol it'll be damaging other organs in your body as well as your liver, and it will definitely be affecting your blood pressure and your heart. Just in case you need more incentive to cut down, excessive alcohol increases your risk of some cancers such as cancers of the mouth and throat, and unfortunately liver disease is often symptomless until it's far advanced. The more people drink from a younger age, the more likely they'll be to have health problems.

Alcoholic drinks are full of hidden calories. Look at IDEA 11, *Battle of the bulge*, on ways to control your weight.

Try another idea...

There is some good news, though. Drinking one to two units of alcohol a day does help to protect you against heart disease if you're already at the risk of it: say, if you're a man over forty or a woman after the menopause. Despite what you may hear, this is any alcohol and not just red wine. A small amount of alcohol helps to lower levels of 'bad' cholesterol that would fur up your arteries otherwise. It also makes your blood less sticky and less likely to clot.

Ah, but... you knew there had to be a but, didn't you? Drinking *more* than one or two units every day gradually reduces the health benefits. When you drink as much as the recommended daily limits the benefits to your heart are outweighed by the harm you are doing to other parts of your body. It's all about balance. By the way, you don't have to start drinking red wine or whatever to protect your heart, if you don't want to, because even a small amount of regular alcohol can increase the risks of cancer and cirrhosis.

'My wife suggested I cut back by a glass of claret per day. I was so impressed, I opened a bottle to toast her.'
FREDERICK FORSYTH, British author

Defining idea...

Q **Is alcohol good for me even though I've had a heart attack?**

A *Yes, it can be. It even seems to help straight after a heart attack when the blood supply to your heart is being re-established.*

Q **I love to go out for a glass. I'd be a miserable sod without it and that would be bad for me... So how can I cut down?**

A *If you get so much pleasure drinking in company, reserve the alcohol you allow yourself for when you're out; don't drink alone at home. Go out a bit later so you won't spend as much time at the bar. Keep count and alternate alcoholic drinks with soft drinks; you could top up with lots of mixers. Pace yourself: drink more slowly by timing yourself, sipping that first one, perhaps playing games like pool with your friends while having a drink. Eat before you drink and eat while you drink – that should help you to slow down. If anyone tries to persuade you to drink more, refuse. Enjoy your friends' company, laugh and chat – fun doesn't depend on how much alcohol you can get down you.*

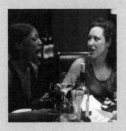 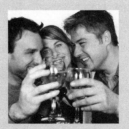

24

Mind out

If you're feeling anxious or depressed you're more likely to bring on heart disease. Change your outlook on life and your heart will thank you.

Anxiety, panic disorder and depression are common in people who suffer from heart disease or raised blood pressure; if untreated, their heart disease can become worse. So it's time for help.

DESPAIRS is a mnemonic that lists the symptoms of depression. If you've got the first of these plus at least four of the others, then that's it, you're definitely depressed. No need for a psychiatrist, fancy tests or state-of-the-art equipment – this simple mnemonic diagnoses you:

- Depressed mood or disinterest in your usual activities;
- Energy loss or tiredness;
- Sleep disturbance;
- Pessimism or hopelessness;
- Appetite and weight change;
- Impaired concentration or inability to remember things;

Here's an idea for you...

Write a list of all the good things in your life on a card and get it laminated. Stick it on the front of your wardrobe to remind you that life is good when you get up in the morning and go to bed at night. Stick a copy on the fridge door or on a mirror downstairs as a memo. Then you'll see that even if there are things happening in your life to make you sad, it's only natural and they're counterbalanced by the good things anyway. If you've had a heart attack, then maybe you're grieving for the loss of your health or fitness, but there are still loads of things you can do.

- Retardation or agitation;
- Suicidal ideas or recurrent thoughts of death.

If you tend to have depression and anxiety, then you're more likely to have heart disease and increased blood pressure too. If you've already got heart disease and become depressed, you're more likely to go on to suffer a fatal heart attack; in fact you're three or four times more likely to do so than if you were feeling fine mentally. If you're depressed, you may even have more side effects and worse symptoms from the drugs doctors give you to treat your heart or blood pressure. And depression is a double whammy: you won't be as determined to change your lifestyle for the better and stick to stopping smoking or taking regular exercise. You won't be bothered, may feel too tired and be generally uninterested in boosting your health.

The trouble is that the drugs you take for your heart disease or blood pressure may clash with any drug treatments for your depression or anxiety. Some of the newer drugs on the market are safer for you when you've got heart disease than the older anti-depressants were. Being on the newer drugs increases your chances of survival if you were to have a heart attack while still depressed.

Anti-depressants don't work immediately and it can be quite a few weeks before the benefits kick in. If you stop too soon taking them you might relapse, so once you've started and they're working keep going for six to twelve months. The older you are, the longer you might take them for. St John's Wort is often said to be good for mild depression, but if you're on heart drugs like digoxin or warfarin it can interact with them – don't assume that just because it is a herbal medicine it's harmless; it's a powerful substance, after all.

Remember that exercise is one of the most effective treatments for depression and get those walking boots on – take the first step with IDEA 5, *Step outside*.

Try another idea...

Acupuncture can help your depression. So can psychotherapy – so make time for talking yourself better. Music probably helps too; there's no particular kind to recommend more than another, you've not got to develop a new taste for classical or rock music. And it might work better if you do art therapy, or have massage, or visualise happy scenes at the same time. Yoga and relaxation are other kinds of treatments that can help depression. Most of these treatments for depression help anxiety too; this isn't surprising as they often coexist. Kava kava is worth a try if you're suffering from anxiety or panic attacks. Take 300 mg per day, divided up as several doses. And don't forget that counselling may well help; this could be a community psychiatric nurse or psychologist, or just a sensible friend, someone to tell your troubles to, who listens with interest to all the small details of your life. And the more your depression lifts, the better for your heart.

'Any man who goes to a psychiatrist should have his head examined.'
SAM GOLDWYN, film director

Defining idea...

How did it go?

Q **I have been depressed for ages but I am frightened of getting addicted to anti-depressants so I have refused to take them. How addictive are they?**

A *Nowadays most antidepressants are not addictive. But once you've taken an antidepressant for more than a few weeks, and when it's time to discontinue them, you should gradually taper off the dose you take each day to avoid any reaction from stopping too quickly. Otherwise you might get flu-like withdrawal symptoms including dizziness, nausea, tingling, headache, tremor, palpitations and anxiety – just what you were trying to treat.*

Q **Sometimes I think I'm having a heart attack. My heart beats so fast that I start gulping for air thinking I'm going to suffocate and my hands tingle. What's going on?**

A *Sounds like you're 'over-breathing', part of having a panic attack. If you recognise you're doing this, slow your breathing down by consciously counting yourself breathing in and out once, over about five seconds. You can breathe into a paper bag or your cupped hands, covering your nose and mouth, for three to five minutes. This will mean you're re-breathing old air and cutting down the amount of oxygen you're inhaling after all your over-breathing. Take your mind off the panic attack by distracting yourself with what else is going on around you. Learn to make yourself relax your muscles in sequence, clenching your hands and arms then working along to your neck, chest, stomach, buttocks and legs.*

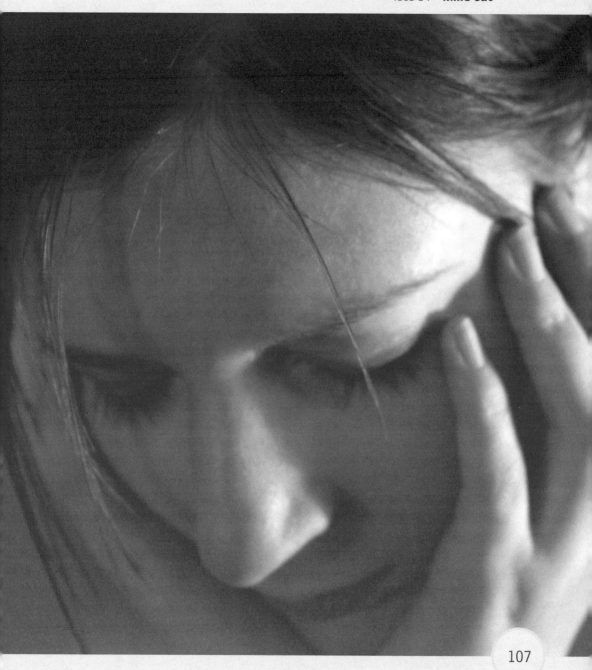

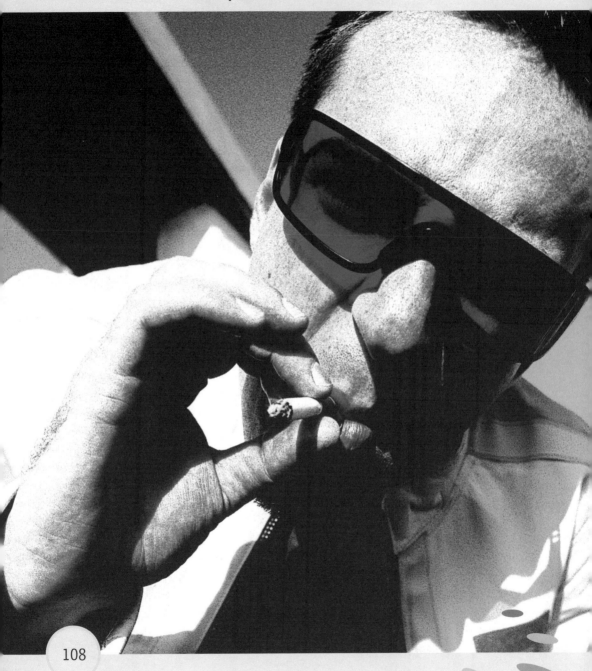

25

Break with stress

Are you a control freak? If not, maybe you should be, as that's the best way to beat stress – get control over your work or problems, cut the demands on you.

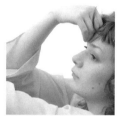

There's 'good' stress and 'bad' stress, though. With 'good' stress you enjoy the challenge, you bask in your hard-won achievements. With 'bad' stress, the demands on you are too much for you to cope with and you suffer for it.

It looks as if stress, combined with other risk factors for heart disease – like smoking and having a high cholesterol level – can cause heart disease or make it worse. Stress doesn't happen in a vacuum. Pressures and problems at home often overflow into how you feel and perform at work, and the effects of stress at work are often taken home and dumped there.

You know that if you're under stress, your heart pounds and you can even get palpitations. It sometimes feels as if your heart is going to burst and that people nearby have got to be able to hear your heart thumping away, it's so loud. When you meet a challenge or a threat, your body clicks into a 'fight or flight' mode, ready for action. Adrenaline and cortisol surge through your bloodstream, getting

Here's an idea for you...

Keep a stress log for a few weeks. Carry a pocket-sized diary with you, or run up some diary sheets on your notebook computer. Note down anything that causes you stress, whether you're at work, home or out with your mates. If you've time, record how you reacted. Just a few key words will do. Then at the end of the day, or every few days, look at your notes to see if there's a pattern. Discuss these with a friend or your partner. Plan to avoid or cut out the things that are causing you stress as far as you can.

you ready to run away or stand and fight. It's a pity that it's such a useless reaction for most stresses of modern life; you just get the side effects – increased blood pressure and stirred-up fatty deposits in your arteries. Being stressed can lead to some bad habits, too, ones which put more strain on your heart. You might eat for comfort, drink alcohol to drown your sorrows, maybe give up exercise because you no longer care about keeping fit.

There are as many checklists for telling you if you're stressed as there are minutes in a decade. So I'm not going to waste space reproducing one of them – anyway, you already know the feeling: sweaty, heart pounding, dry mouth, headaches, losing interest in hobbies or work, going off sex, losing your appetite, being tearful, feeling tired, etc., etc. These are all symptoms of stress, you don't need a chart to tell you that. What you want to know is how to deal with it, not get more stressed just reading about it.

The key is to learn how you must deal with pressure if you want to beat stress. You're lucky if your personality is upbeat and optimistic: then you'll keep a positive attitude instead of getting angry or depressed. Pessimists, please note: you've got to try and develop a positive mantra – keep repeating nice words about yourself, dwell on good things about your life. Consider what life events are going on around you.

Well, if you're going through a divorce, have just lost your mum, have moved house or lost a job, it's no wonder you feel down or stressed: you're just reacting as anyone would, so don't expect too much of yourself. That way you just add extra stress.

To discover other sources of information and help, check out IDEA 44, *A heart-warming read.*

Try another idea...

Preventing things from getting too bad is the best form of stress management – the earlier you act, the better. So spot the stress and try to do something to avoid it happening. Stress-proofing is what you need, so make time and space for yourself: for fun, relaxation, hobbies and enjoying simple pleasures. Limit your workload so that you can enjoy a life outside work, and factor in enough time for having fun. Find methods of relaxation that work for you. Follow a healthy lifestyle – eating healthy foods, taking regular exercise, not smoking, limiting the amount of alcohol you drink – and look after your health. You need time for rest and recuperation like anyone else.

Then, talk things through. Even if it's not in your nature to confide in other people, talk about your worries to others, maybe those at work who are responsible for the stress you're under or who are able to alleviate it. Seek the support of your colleagues, friends and family. You'll feel better telling someone about your problems, and they may have ideas too to help reduce the sources of stress that are bugging you.

'What is this life if, full of care, We have no time to stand and stare?'
WILLIAM DAVIES, poet

Defining idea...

How did it go?

Q I don't have anyone to confide in about how stressed I am. My boss is a right tyrant; he causes a lot of my stress and my wife won't listen. What can I do?

A   *It can be difficult, but you've got to stand up to your boss, and woo your wife to get her on your side. Can you go to your trade union about your boss, or your personnel department? Or get the others at work to sort things out with you, so it's not all falling on you? Once you start taking action you'll feel a bit better. Promise.*

Q It's all very well telling me to relax – how can I with a full-time job and a family to cope with?

A   *Learn to make the most of any free period, even just a few minutes. Try and train yourself to shut right off from your surroundings. At work, lock yourself in the loo for five minutes or sit in your car at lunchtime. At home, there's always the garden shed...*

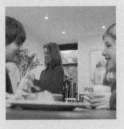
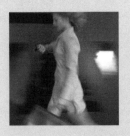

26

Sleep, glorious sleep

Do you have an impossible dream of going to sleep at ten and waking at seven the next morning?

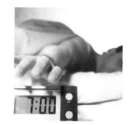

A good restful sleep is vital to your physical and emotional well-being, so it's time to put the lid on insomnia.

If your sleep is disturbed, you'll feel irritable and down next day, and find it difficult to concentrate at work. Ultimately your heart will suffer.

Are you doing anything which is obviously keeping you awake, like drinking too much coffee? You could switch to decaffeinated drinks or other alternatives. Substitute redbush tea, or herbal teas (without liquorice) for a change. If it's alcohol or other stimulants that are stopping you from dropping off, then cut them out. Try eating regularly during the day and avoid having a heavy meal late at night – or your stomach churning will keep you awake.

Maybe painful joints are keeping you awake? You could take painkillers just before you climb into bed, or get the cause seen to. Is your bed uncomfortable? Well, buy a firmer mattress, or put a board under your existing one. Is the bed long enough or do your feet hang out over the end? Try more covers on the bed to keep you warm

You'll sleep better with exercise. Being tired might seem essential to promoting good sleep, but it doesn't necessarily work like that; you can lie staring at the ceiling for ages. It's got to be the right sort of tired, exhaustion from physical rather than mental exercise. So get at least four to six hours of moderate exercise a week and your sleep should improve. That's only a matter of a fifteen-minute walk a day in the morning and again in the evening with a few more trips up and down the stairs.

'Laugh and the world laughs with you; snore and you sleep alone.'
ANTHONY BURGESS, British author

or get lighter ones if you're overheating. Make sure the room's dark enough for you; some people sleep a lot better if they've got blackout curtains, so that dawn doesn't wake them too early.

You could be mulling things over in your mind. Anxiety and worry are terrible for keeping you awake and stopping you from dropping off. Or maybe it's depression? If so, you'll probably be waking early, around 4 a.m., and catnapping, finding it difficult to get back to a proper sleep. You could be worrying about your finances or feeling stressed from work or your everyday life. Think your problems through, make plans for dealing with them – and then set them aside. Visualise yourself placing your problems in a box and closing the lid on them, so you'll drop off to sleep unworried.

Keep a sleep diary. Once you know what's causing you to lose sleep, you can tackle the source and hopefully sleep better for it. You might also want to try some relaxation techniques. Move through a simple relaxing sequence before getting into bed. Finish work earlier, read quietly, or do some yoga. Have a hot bath and wallow in it. Learn to switch off mentally when you turn off the light; picture a pleasant scene where you're relaxed, not one

Some herbal medicines can help you to sleep better; look at IDEA 19, *Herbs-enlist*, for more on them.

Try another idea...

that will start getting you fired up by thinking of the new experiences you might have there or replaying old troubles. Other relaxation techniques like autogenic training, biofeedback and meditation could help you drop off and sleep better. Hypnotherapy might work for you to improve your sleep. T'ai chi may help you relax, too. You might want to try melatonin – taken in the evening, this should help you fall asleep, and if taken in the morning, should prolong sleep.

Finally, don't forget to keep it quiet. Move to another bedroom, if you can, if traffic noise keeps you awake. If you've a noisy partner, you could always wear ear plugs or get them to try snoring aids!

Q **My restless legs give me horrible sensations when I'm lying in bed, like insects crawling on me and electric currents tingling. How can I sleep better?**

How did it go?

A *You're more likely to get restless legs syndrome (RLS) as you get older, or if you're overweight. Take regular exercise and do all the other sensible lifestyle things. Try rubbing your legs or having a hot bath before you go to bed to boost your circulation. There's always the option to go to your doctor for drug treatment if these things don't work.*

115

Q   I've tried everything but when I go to bed I just lie awake for hours. Now what?

A   *Only go to bed when you feel sleepy. If you've been there for twenty minutes or so without dropping off to sleep, then get up and do a non-stimulating activity in another room, maybe reading something light or listening to music (listening to soothing music before bedtime can also improve your sleep quality). Still get up at the same time in the morning whatever time you got off to sleep, so you establish a regular habit. That'll condition you to associate being in bed with being asleep.*

Q   What about sleeping tablets? Are they OK to take if you've got heart disease?

A   *There are drugs you can take if you must. Some, like zopiclone, stay in your body for a much shorter period than drugs like benzodiazepines, so you're less likely to have hangover sleepiness next day. It's easy to get addicted, so only take them on two or three nights a week and for a few consecutive nights every so often: otherwise you won't sleep with them and you won't be able to sleep without them, either. Give homeopathic drugs such as aconite, lycopodium or sulphur a try instead. You'll take them during the evening, repeat the dose at bedtime and possibly during the night if necessary.*

27

Health at work

You want promotion at work so you earn more – but what about health promotion, so you learn more and live longer with your healthy heart?

It makes good business sense for organisations to invest in helping staff to be more healthy. The more they do for their staff, the less sick leave they'll take, and the happier the team will be.

Check out your workplace for what's being done to encourage you all to take more exercise. There'll be bicycle racks outside, and showers in the washrooms to encourage people to cycle into work, in the most health-conscious organisations; your company could do these things too. And it's not just encouraging cycling: there are lots of other benefits your company could arrange – like a reduced subscription to a local gym. It won't cost them anything, as the gym will offer price cuts for the mass recruitment they hope to get out of such a scheme.

More informally, find some kindred spirits. Get a group of exercise nuts together for regular power walks at lunchtime; a thirty-minute walk at more than four miles an hour will get your day's quota of exercise done. And the bonus is that there's less

Here's an idea for you... **Set up a health library at your workplace. Include books, videos, CDs and posters you can plaster on corridors or office walls. Borrow videos or CDs on exercise routines and give them a go. There could be cook books on low-fat cooking, perhaps, or information pamphlets to help smokers wanting to quit. Perhaps posters could advertise healthy themes or activities you're going to run for groups of staff? Don't forget to include frequently asked questions – and some answers, giving other people's tips.**

time for eating and drinking! The downside is less time for gossip and news; you won't be able to chat much while you power along. And what about a sports league? Can you play sport on your work premises or at a club nearby? Don't just think team sports like football, but also things like badminton or squash, or even table tennis. All of these will bring great benefits, quite apart from encouraging health – there'll be improvements in your communal spirit as getting people together with common interests will help the work ethos, too. If your department is health conscious, then they could buy equipment to lend out like stepping machines for people to experiment with and see if they want to buy or rent one themselves. A take-it-yourself blood pressure machine in a corner of the office would allow people to check themselves – who knows, you could even use it to log your blood pressure when stressed by the management...

Now, what about a staff 'awayday' that's centred around activity? Not just one where people are locked in a room ruminating on why things aren't going well: get out in the country on a walk or team exercise, taking a

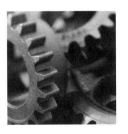

challenge or joining in a group ramble. You could always have a day based round a golf tournament.

Remember your kindred spirits? You all want to lead healthy lifestyles, don't you? You're all human, and weak when it comes to giving up some of your hard-won vices. So get some groups going, maybe to lose weight, quit smoking, take exercise or just have fun. One of you could lead, and weigh or monitor the others. You could involve a company nurse, or a role model who's successfully kicked a bad habit, or just the keen member of staff with a clipboard who organises everyone else. You could have graphs comparing everyone, with a prize for the best or rewards for milestones, or it could be a private affair. You could even have a red-face day where you regularly embarrass people who have strayed from their agreed contract, or you could be more kindly and work in pairs to support each other. Something will suit your group.

You could set up a stress-busting club at work. Look at IDEA 25, *Break with stress*, for the kind of problems you'll be trying to overcome and ways to do it.

Try another idea...

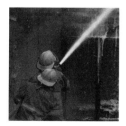

'If A is a success in life, then A equals x plus y plus z. Work is x; y is play; and z is keeping your mouth shut.'
ALBERT EINSTEIN

Defining idea...

Q **I work for a massive company which has an occupational health service. Are we right to be scared of the doctors finding out what's wrong with our health so the management can force us out?**

A   *The doctors and nurses employed by your management, will be briefed to do their best for employees too. Whatever your worries on that score, they should be useful to you to boost how healthy your workplace is. Invite them along to discuss all your plans to improve the health of the staff. Discuss any dangers you've noted – and tell them what equipment you need, too, to be able to lift more safely or perform other work functions, for example.*

Q **Should our workplace have a defibrillator standing by in case anyone has a heart attack and needs resuscitating?**

A   *Why not? So long as someone knows how to use it, and it's the kind that's meant for homes and workplaces, to be used by the general public. It should be easy to use and have a self-checking function that shows it's in working order. It could only be a bonus for you all, just in case. And it's an especially good idea in workplaces where lots of older people are employed.*

Q **Anything else we can do at our workplace to encourage staff to be healthy and work effectively?**

A   *Have you got water machines strategically positioned, so people can get drinking water whenever they want without having to traipse a long way and lose time from their desks? Does someone replace the water when the bottles run dry? What about self-service machines? If staff stay late and do overtime, they'll get hungry; and if you already have them, can people get a healthy snack or is it just crisps and chocolate that're available?*

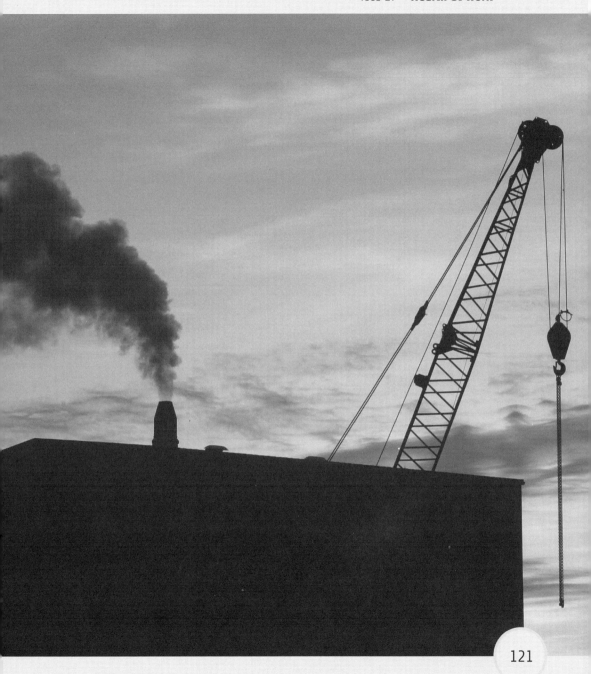

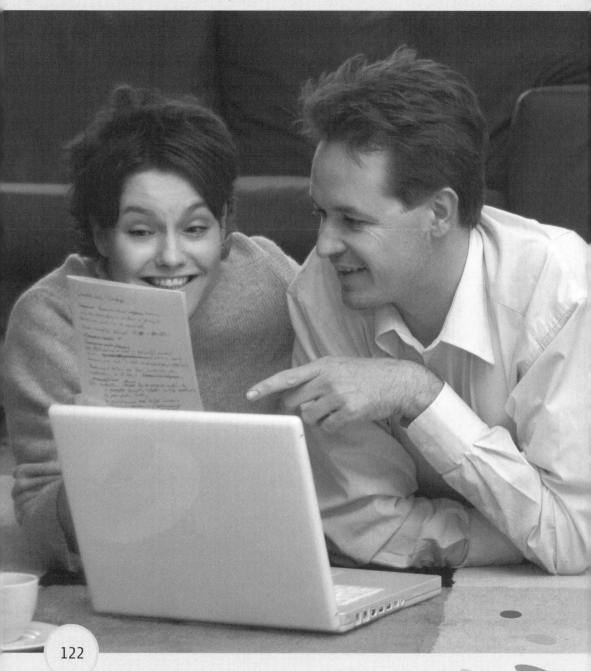

28

Work at it

It's official: job satisfaction is good for your health. Here are some tips to help you get the most out of your work and start enjoying it, for the sake of your heart.

If your heart's not in it, going to work will be a chore and you'll get disillusioned and depressed.

Having a certain prestige in society, as a manager or a professional, actually protects you against heart disease: the more you're in control of the demands made upon you at work, the more you're protected from the effects of stress. On the whole, the further you went in education, the less likely you are to develop heart disease. All of these sort of factors add up to you having more income from a good job: people who have more money coming in tend to have less heart disease. But then they often smoke less, too.

Lots more people believe that work-related stress is making them ill than is probably the case. Certain types of work situations are stressful, of course – especially if you've got lots of work piled on you and you can't control it. You might be having to work long shifts and be deprived of sleep. Maybe your work is dangerous; if you're frightened and in personal danger, that's obviously stressful.

123

See if you can make the most of any opportunities for flexible working. Start and finish earlier, so you've more time with your family or to play sport in after hours. Try a job share with someone else, so you stay in an interesting, responsible job that wouldn't otherwise be possible on a part-time basis. Annualised hours – where you work a certain number of hours or days per year or month – might help you balance your commitments outside work, and help with peak demands at work or the school holidays at home. It could give you more choice and control in your life.

Defining idea...

'And no one shall work for money, and no one shall work for fame, But each for the joy of working.'
RUDYARD KIPLING

If you clash with your managers at work, then they can make your life hell. All these mix together with other causes of heart disease – like having a family history of heart disease, smoking, having high cholesterol – to make matters worse for you. And in addition, the more strain from your job, the more likely you are to eat chocolate and smoke for comfort – and the more difficult it is to quit. So here are some actions you can take.

■ In the long term, get yourself an education and more qualifications so you can get a better job, and you'll be safeguarding your heart. Look at distance-learning possibilities on the internet; enrol for a part-time course. Find out if there's any workplace learning you can do which will lead to promotion and give you transferable skills for a more senior post. Then you'll be the top dog instead of the one taking orders, and you can pace your work in a more orderly way.

■ Once you know that travelling in traffic, either by car or on public transport, almost trebles your risk of a heart attack for at least an hour afterwards, maybe you'll use the phone, email or videoconferencing more often instead. Fumes from car exhausts, road-rage-provoking traffic, noise and the actual stress from travelling all contribute to the strain on your heart. So, yes, cycling to work is good for keeping fit and staying active but bad from the point of view of coping with the effects of traffic. It's a matter of balance.

Learn to control demands on your time, before any excessive pressures affect you adversely. Turn to IDEA 48, *About time*, to read more.

Try another idea...

■ Enjoy your work. Job satisfaction protects you against stress from work. So get in touch with your values and beliefs, then find a job that matches those. See how you fit these eight categories that describe what you no doubt value as being important about your career or job: your competence, management, autonomy and independence, security or stability, creativity, service or dedication to a cause, pure challenge and, finally, your lifestyle. Which of these do you prize most highly and wouldn't give up if you were forced to make a choice? Once you know, try and stick with jobs that match with what you know you value, or you'll lose interest and find you're just going to work for the money. That's often the start of problems.

'Man must work by the sweat of his brow whatever his class, and that should make up the whole meaning and purpose of his life and happiness and contentment.'
ANTON CHEKHOV

Defining idea...

How did it go?

Q **I have to attend lots of business lunches and they're not exactly healthy. How can I resist the specialities of the house?**

A *Just be careful that you don't let your guard slip when you're out with friends or on business. If you drink alcohol, your resolve may crumble and you may have that bread roll or rich pudding after all. Choose low-fat options on the menu, whether or not they're your favourite foods. Keep to it – it'll be worth it in the end.*

Q **I'm a technophobe and want some tips on beating my techno stress before it beats me. What d'you think I can do?**

A *Have plenty of breaks from high-tech gadgets through the day so you get refreshed. Restrict the time you spend on the computer or cell phone by reading or having face-to-face discussions instead. Anticipate a technology crisis by backing up your computer files regularly and limit the time you spend surfing the internet; have some favourite sites to search for information in your field. When you want to concentrate on writing a complex report, take the phone off the hook, turn off the email alert and put a sign on your office door so that you can get on undisturbed.*

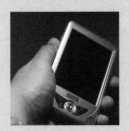

29

Get rich, quick

People who are more affluent have fewer heart problems. So join the rich list by earning more, investing in shares (sharing other people's money) or cutting your losses.

Across the world, people in higher socio-economic groups live several years longer than poorer people. Exactly why is a long story, but there's no doubt about it — so invest in the health of your heart.

Be mercenary if you must. Marry money. This is the quickest way to become rich if you're not going to inherit wealth… and it only takes a few minutes, apart from all the preparatory work, checking out your partner's accounts, interviewing the parents, etc. But then there's also time spent on the search for the appropriate mate – and the expenses of wining and dining, buying the right clothes, and affording membership fees to the right clubs. Do consider long-term earning ability before you plump for the first rich partner to come along and don't forget someone working as a footballer or model has a short shelf-life when you do your financial calculations. But do remember that happy couples live longer than single people. Ah, well…

Here's an idea for you...

Make your spare time work for you. Get paid for your hobby. You could opt for potential money-spinning hobbies like collecting antiques or fine art, or stamp collecting; trainspotting just doesn't cut it in terms of improving your finances.

OK, let's be more serious. Have you got a career plan? Or are you someone whose jobs just happen to come along when you're available to apply for them? You need to develop a mindset where you suck what you can for yourself out of every job you do – all the transferable knowledge and skills you can gain from your current job which will make you ultra-attractive to the next interview panel. Take every developmental opportunity going, up until you retire. The more skills and experience you've got, the more you can diversify and find jobs that suit you so that you're happy at work, and with a lucrative salary to boot. See if there's some career coaching you can get or pay for. You need to be continually looking forward and planning career gains. And if you're thinking of working for yourself, do the sums carefully before you opt for setting up your own business. Remember, there could be lots of hassle and outgoings in terms of staff salaries, office expenses, advertising costs, loss leaders, etc.

Defining idea...

'Those who have some means think that the most important thing in the world is love. The poor know that it is money.'
GERALD BRENAN, author

Then boost your pension. You'll want to be able to retire when you want to, with enough income to be comfortable (and ward off heart disease – yes, really, though no one's quite sure how that works). So start saving for your future now by maximising any pension contributions you can make. Make an informed decision to transfer pensions from your previous posts to your new job if that's possible or in your personal interest. If you moonlight outside your regular job, then make private pension contributions from that if possible. If you're entirely self-employed, then take good advice from an unbiased financial adviser. See if you're better off making private pension contributions or perhaps investing in property to rent out to other people as a pseudo-pension. You'll need to take the hassle factor into account here too: is the extra income worth troublesome tenants or maintenance problems?

Remember that work isn't everything. Look at IDEA 37, *Have fun*, for ways to incorporate more fun into your life.

Try another idea…

Finally, don't forget to cut your expenditure. If you limit any wasteful spending, then you'll have more core income, and that will make you feel more affluent – definitely a happy state for your heart. So if you worry about your finances, aim to spend 80–90% of your income, not the 110% which means always being in debt. Then you'll always feel well off. Substitute cheaper holidays for long-haul ones, buy a sensible car rather than a flashy model, make clothes last several years instead of discarding them after a few months. There really is a lot you can do, quite apart from bagging that supermodel or footballer…

'The main value of money is not to have to do things you don't want to do and to be able to do the things you do want to do. It's a means to a way of living.'
EDWARD DE BONO, writer and lateral thinker

Defining idea…

Q **There are few career opportunities in the small town where I live and it's a long drive otherwise. What can someone like me do?**

A *Hmm. You've got to think more widely. With the internet, fax, phone, a webcam or video link, you can work productively from any location, however far-flung. You just need the ideas – then maybe qualifications and some experience. So think about what kind of retraining you could do. The drive you need is your internal push, not the long and winding road kind.*

Q **Can having money *really* buy you more time before you die?**

A *It certainly looks as though it can. All the statistics show that richer people in the Western world live on average an extra six or seven years than their poorer compatriots. Of course, it depends on what you spend your money on. If it's drugs and fast living, then you'd be lucky to live to an old age, but if money gives you security, good nutrition, a safe job, healthy surroundings and pastimes, then the dice is loaded in your favour.*

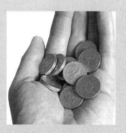
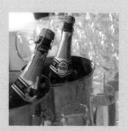

30

Act in time

If someone collapses and their heart stops, it could be up to you to do basic life support. Every second counts.

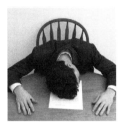

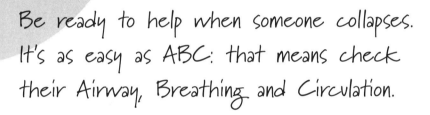

Be ready to help when someone collapses. It's as easy as ABC: that means check their Airway, Breathing and Circulation.

SO KNOW YOUR ABC

Phone the emergency services or get someone to a hospital right away if they have chest pain or discomfort, are short of breath, are in a cold sweat and seem to be having a heart attack. Suspect pain radiating from the chest to both arms, to the neck, jaw or stomach. If they've collapsed, buy time until help arrives by having a go at resuscitating them. You can't let someone lie there with no circulation, or they'll have irreversible brain damage.

Look about you. First, consider if you're safe where you are. Is there live electricity nearby or in contact with the casualty? Don't risk your safety in the middle of a busy road or on a precarious ledge; pull the person to a safer position before you start. OK, you know not to move someone if it's possible that they're unconscious, but weigh up the dangers. If it's no contest, then stay safe: pull them out of danger.

Here's an idea for you...

If you or a relative have had a heart attack in the past, consider buying a home defibrillator as a standby, and make sure there's someone around who could operate it. The home defibrillator can be used by virtually any ordinary person with less than an hour's training. One example of this kind (check out www.brompton.net) provides clear voice instructions that guide the user through every step of the defibrillation process. The defibrillator is a similar size and weight to a hardback book and does its own self-tests each day to ensure it's maintained and ready. The battery lasts for up to four years.

Try to get a response. Shout a command in an authoritative way. Squeeze their shoulders. Look into their mouth and check there are no foreign bodies. Place two fingers under the chin and put your other hand on their forehead, to push it back and extend and straighten the airway. Check if you can feel or hear their breathing for ten seconds, or if you can see their chest move as they breathe.

Still no luck? Then you'll have to start ventilating them. Seal your mouth over theirs while you continue to tip their head backwards and elevate their chin. Then blow into their mouth for two seconds, rest for four seconds and do it again. Check that their chest is rising and falling as you blow into their lungs.

Still no joy? They're not breathing by themselves? There's no sign of life? Check for a pulse in their neck or elsewhere – their wrist or heart. If there isn't one, you'll have to start doing chest compressions. Place the heel of your hand over the lower part of their breastbone, the width of two fingers above where the ribs join together. Keep your arms straight and use the weight of your body to press down. Aim to compress the chest by 4–5 cm, making fifteen compressions in quick sequence within about ten seconds. Continue to switch between giving two breaths and fifteen compressions until professional help arrives, or you see signs of life, or you're just too exhausted to carry on.

We all spend so much time at work that you might want to suggest having a defibrillator there. Check out IDEA 27, *Health at work*, for more helpful suggestions.

Try another idea...

WHAT A DEFIBRILLATOR CAN DO

If the person's heart has stopped, it can be restarted with an electric shock given by a defibrillator. Two-thirds of people who have a cardiac arrest have an over-fast heart rhythm – ventricular fibrillation, or tachycardia – which can revert to normal with an electric charge from a defibrillation machine, if this is given quickly enough. These days you may be able or expected to use a defibrillator even if you're not a doctor or nurse. Automatic defibrillators are increasingly sited in public places such as supermarkets, shopping centres, train stations and aircraft.

A defibrillator discharges a fixed, high-voltage, direct current through pads attached to the person's chest. If there's a defibrillator standing by and it's down to you to use it, connect the leads to the pads before placing the pads on the bare chest, and don't put the pads over jewellery or you might cause a burn. When you press the button, no one should be in physical contact with the person or anything attached to them. If there's no response, try again, giving a maximum of three shocks.

'In the midst of life we are in death.'
The Book of Common Prayer

Defining idea...

133

How did it go?

Q **If someone's collapsed, do I just look into their mouth before starting or should I have a feel inside?**

A *Yes, you should, but have a good look too. When feeling, be careful: don't sweep your finger around as you might dislodge something and push it down further. And leave well-fitting dentures in place.*

Q **I don't really like putting my lips to the mouth of someone I don't know; it seems a bit intimate. What's the alternative?**

A *You could always get a key ring that carries a compact ventilation mask or keep a pocket-sized mask in the first aid kit in your car, office or home. Failing that, you could put a cotton or even paper handkerchief between your mouth and theirs. This will reduce the chances of you getting their saliva or vomit in your mouth while you're trying to resuscitate them. No one's been known to have caught HIV or the hepatitis B virus during mouth-to-mouth ventilation, mind.*

Q **Any special precautions I should take when releasing the defibrillator charge, apart from not touching the person I'm using it on?**

A *If you are in a wet environment make sure there's no water linking the person who has collapsed to your feet, or the electric charge you use to shock the person may be conveyed to you too.*

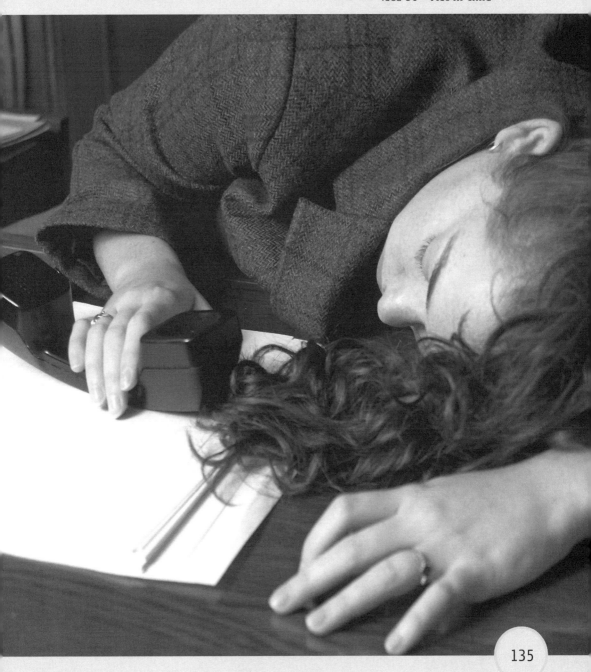

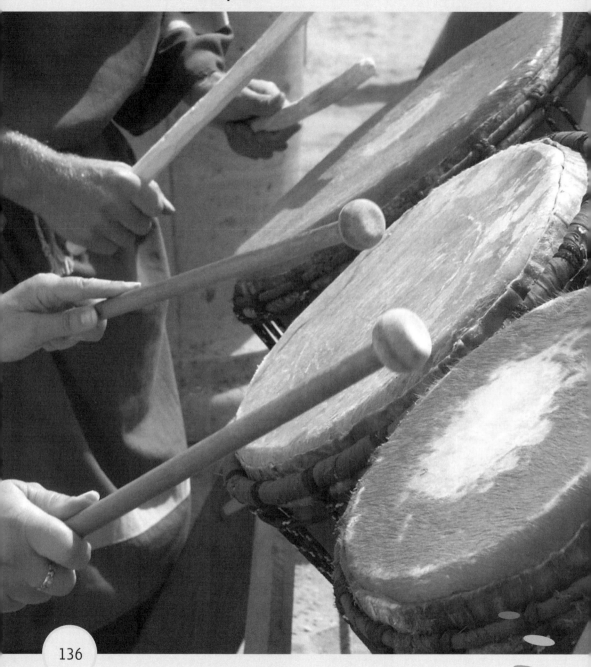

31

Failing that

Heart failure's not about your heart missing a beat when someone jumps out on you unexpectedly. The outlook for heart failure's worse than for many cancers. So it pays to know your enemy.

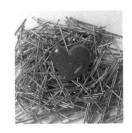

Heart failure sounds serious, and it is. About half the people newly diagnosed with serious heart failure do not survive a year, and about 10% die off every year thereafter.

SO WHAT IS IT?

When your heart beats, it pumps blood around your body. When you've got heart failure, your heart doesn't pump the blood round so well. This means it doesn't supply enough oxygen for your body's needs, especially when you're on the move or exercising. About 10 million people in Europe suffer from heart failure. There's more of it about than there was because people live longer now.

Heart failure occurs when your heart muscle becomes damaged, often after a heart attack when it's less efficient, or if you've got high blood pressure. Sometimes it comes about because of a diseased heart muscle or valve. A rapid heartbeat for some time can lead to heart failure, and so can too much alcohol and some drugs.

Here's an idea for you... **If you've got heart failure, a flu jab every autumn will guard against you getting a dose of influenza which could make you really poorly. Vaccination against pneumococcal disease is another immunisation you can have too, on a one-off basis.**

The clues that you've got it are always being short of breath, especially if you're walking or climbing stairs; having swollen feet or ankles, and tiredness or weakness. Being short of breath can be worse, too, when you lie flat – so bad that you wake up at night. When heart failure begins, maybe after a heart attack, it's often quite sudden. But you could also have chronic heart failure, which can creep up on you.

It's best if anybody suspected of having heart failure has an echocardiogram; that's the 'gold standard' investigation for it. The ultrasound of your heart shows its structure and how it's working, and allows doctors to measure the pressures in it. Lots of people have shortness of breath, and if you don't have an echocardiogram you won't know if you're the one in five who has heart failure out of all of those with shortness of breath. Just going on your symptoms, or what signs doctors can detect by listening to your chest and looking at your body, is unreliable. A heart tracing or electrocardiogram (ECG) may also give the clue – as anyone with a totally normal ECG is unlikely to have heart failure. There's a blood test, too, for b-type natriuretic peptide (BNP) that helps to tell if your symptoms are due to heart failure. This is a naturally occurring hormone that aids heart function and when your heart cannot pump blood efficiently, BNP is produced to help ease its workload.

TREATMENTS

You have to follow all the usual advice for a cardio-friendly diet and lifestyle. It really is best to keep active, even if it's difficult and you don't feel like it and exercising makes you puff. You'll be given a drug – or a mix of drugs – like diuretics (water tablets) to help your body get rid of excess water, ACE inhibitors to relax your blood vessels so that your heart can pump blood more easily through them, beta-blockers to slow your heart rate and reduce the amount of work your heart does, and digoxin to help your heart beat more strongly. Some people will also be taking drugs to thin their blood and guard against clots. By the way, some drugs – like anti-inflammatories for swollen or painful joints – make heart failure worse, so you're best not taking them. Talk to your doctor.

Too much salt can increase your blood pressure and make heart failure worse. So see IDEA 14, *Salt away*, for more tips on ways to reduce the amount of salt in your diet.

Try another idea...

Now, although water tablets will make you thirsty, don't drink too much – keep your fluid intake down to about one and a half to two litres a day – and this means limiting the alcohol you drink, too. Sorry, but alcohol makes heart failure worse, so you're best avoiding it altogether. Anyway, you are supposed to be following a cardio-friendly lifestyle! (By the way, and it's early days, but research has shown that Viagra, the drug for impotence, can reverse heart failure in mice...)

There are some surgical options. If your heart disease is caused by valvular heart disease you might have an operation to replace your heart valve. Sometimes a pacemaker can help or a defibrillator can be implanted under the skin in case you have a life-threatening heart rhythm. A heart transplant is the ultimate surgery – but hopefully that will not be necessary.

'The abbreviation of time, and the failure of hope, will always tinge with a browner shade the evening of life.'
EDWARD GIBBON, British historian

Defining idea...

How did
it go?

Q My gran has heart failure and really can't do anything for herself without getting puffed. What can I do?

A   As well as caring for her, look after yourself as much as you can. You won't be able to help if you make yourself ill, and caring for someone with heart failure can be very demanding. So get regular breaks as often as possible. See if there are volunteers who'll sit with your gran and organise a rota for all the family to take turns doing the caring.

Q Is it true you can have a machine to help your heart to do the pumping if you've got heart failure?

A   Yes, they're called ventricular assist devices. That's where the machine is implanted into your abdomen to support the left ventricle, the main pumping chamber of your heart, or both the right and left ventricles. These devices are sometimes used in really sick people waiting for heart transplants and are powered by rechargeable batteries. Occasionally, the machine buys time for someone's heart to recover from what caused the heart failure, and they no longer need the transplant or eventually, the machine.

32

Tick off

Does your ticker go bump in the night? Or have you just met your heart-throb in the flesh? Hearts doing funny things occasionally can be normal. Hearts doing funny things frequently is not.

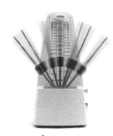

You may just be overly aware of your own normal heartbeat, like when you're waiting for an interview, or maybe a row, to start. If you've got persistent or troublesome palpitations, then specialist treatment should control them.

If you're aware of your heartbeat, then you're experiencing palpitations. Your heart might be beating normally, or quickly, or slowly or irregularly. Or it might be missing beats every so often. Most palpitations are harmless. They can last for a few seconds or minutes or several hours. They're a normal part of the way your body responds to fear, anger and physical activity, and if you've a fever you know that your heart beats faster than usual. When you're aware of your heart beating loudly you think that other people must be able to hear it too, but basically you feel fine. If you were to put a hand on the left side of your chest wall or on the pulse at your wrist you'd notice that your heart was beating fast and regularly, perhaps more than 100 beats per minute compared to your normal 60–80 beats per minute or so.

Here's an idea for you...

Cutting down on coffee is a first step to take in order to be rid of palpitations. Caffeine is a mild stimulant which increases the rate at which your body's metabolism ticks over when adrenaline is released into your bloodstream. Your cup of coffee may make you feel alert, full of energy and ready for action – but all this can make your heart beat faster and palpitations seem worse. So switch to decaffeinated coffee and tea and other drinks, and see if your palpitations improve.

But sometimes palpitations are a sign of heart disease. While you're having them, they might make you sweat or feel faint or dizzy, and you might get chest pains at the same time as the palpitations with lots of extra beats or missed ones. An electrocardiogram (ECG) will help to find out what's going on by recording the electrical activity of your heart. You'll have small sticky patches or electrodes put on your arms, legs and chest and connected to a recording machine which registers the electrical signals produced by your heartbeats. This monitors how fast and regular your heart rate is, as well as looking for any signs of a heart attack, whether your heart has become enlarged or is working under strain. Sometimes an ECG is done while you're exercising on a treadmill or stationary bike instead of lying down resting, to see if exercise triggers your heart to beat in an odd way or show signs of strain.

One common type of very fast and irregular palpitations is atrial fibrillation. About one in twenty-five people over the age of sixty-five experience this. Episodes of atrial fibrillation can last for a few minutes, or hours, or days – or become permanent. Sometimes atrial fibrillation is caused by an overactive thyroid gland, sometimes by high blood pressure, lung infections or heart disease. Sometimes it's a legacy from having had rheumatic fever or heart murmurs as a child. Drinking too much alcohol over time can cause atrial fibrillation, too. If you've had one or more episodes of atrial fibrillation, then you'll probably have had your thyroid gland function tested, had an ECG and maybe an echocardiogram as well to assess how your heart valves are functioning and check on the size and structure of your heart. Having atrial fibrillation does increase your risk of stroke, heart failure and dying prematurely. That's why one of the treatments is to thin your blood with the drug warfarin, making it less likely for clots to form in your bloodstream and trigger a heart attack or stroke. Whether you're advised to take warfarin or aspirin depends on your calculated level of risk of a stroke versus the likely benefits to you of treatment and possible disadvantages, like causing your gut to bleed.

Too much alcohol is another trigger for palpitations. Check out IDEA 23, *Booze over*, for more information.

Try another idea...

There are drugs that can control a too-fast heart rate. If they don't work, then cardioversion – an electric shock given under general anaesthetic – may do the trick. Another method is to use radio frequency energy to ablate or destroy the abnormal part of the electrical pathway in your heart which is causing the atrial fibrillation rhythm. An artificial pacemaker is yet another treatment choice; your doctor will explain what's right for you.

'"Madame café, I am your slave," said the man. "You make my hands shake, my knees quake, my heart beat. Oh my sweet."'
Wall poster in the Eden Project, UK

Defining idea...

143

How did it go?

Q **I'm under loads of stress at work so I get palpitations a lot and don't know if they're normal. What can I do?**

A *Well, one way to let a doctor know what your palpitations are like is to beat out the rhythm and timing on a table with your fingers – any past experience of drumming may come in handy here. Your doctor can arrange for you to have an ECG and if that's normal and you've no other symptoms, will probably reassure you that your palpitations are a normal reaction to stress. Start looking at job ads and see what other work's available.*

Q **Do I get palpitations! They'll suddenly come on, making me gasp for breath, sweat and feel faint. Like I'm choking, and I'm nauseated with a dry mouth. They say these are panic attacks, but how do I cope with them?**

A *Panic attacks are not harmful or dangerous. They're just an exaggeration of your normal bodily response to stress and nothing worse than those feelings is going to happen. Just take a deep breath; slow down your breathing pattern. Distract yourself by thinking of something different. Give the fear time to pass and the palpitations should gradually subside.*

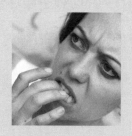 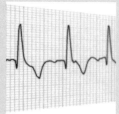

33

It's a pain

Having to live with angina is a complete pain, but there's lots you can do for it.

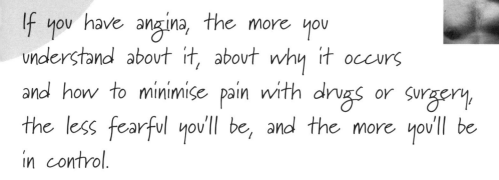

If you have angina, the more you understand about it, about why it occurs and how to minimise pain with drugs or surgery, the less fearful you'll be, and the more you'll be in control.

Angina is an uncomfortable feeling in your chest, one that you'd describe as heaviness or tightness, or maybe just as pain or an ache. It can spread from the centre of your chest to your arm (your left more than the right), neck, jaw, back or stomach, or – unusually – your throat. It might bypass your chest and go straight to your arm, neck, stomach or jaw.

The pain comes on when you exert yourself or get upset or are outside in the cold. When you stop exerting yourself or come in, the pain usually fades and stops. Having a tablet or squirt of glyceryl trinitrate (GTN) helps to relieve angina pain more quickly than if you just wait for it to subside. If your chest pain is bad, does

Here's an idea for you...

Destress yourself to keep your angina away. Try scoring the sources of stress in your life with a traffic-light system. A red light means devastating stress, like a family rift, so try to avoid these from occurring. With an amber light you must minimise the impact of the stress or how frequently it happens, something like being late for work. Green light stress can be challenging and boost your spirits so long as it's in moderation – like being competitive at your favourite sport – but too much will make you feel pressured.

not go away when you stop and rest, and you're sweating or feel sick or breathless, then you may be having a heart attack. So get medical help urgently and get to hospital straight away.

Your doctor will decide, with you, if you're better taking one or more drugs to prevent the angina pain coming on, or if you should just take a quick dose of GTN when your pain starts. They'll use a 'stepwise' approach with you, introducing different and stronger drugs if the first ones don't control your angina pain, or give you side effects.

If you can predict that your chest pain will come on with exercise and is controlled by drugs, then it's called *stable* angina. If it's *unstable,* then either it has just developed, or it's got worse or changed its pattern, or the pain is just carrying on for perhaps more than twenty minutes even though you're resting. If you've got unstable angina and your chest pain's escalating, you'll need to be admitted to hospital as an emergency and monitored to see if you need anti-clotting drugs, strong pain killers, aspirin, etc. The whole idea is to stop any damage caused by a clot breaking off the wall of one of the arteries in your heart, and triggering or worsening a heart attack.

An exercise ECG is done while you're using a treadmill or an exercise bike, with you attached to the ECG's electrical leads to investigate your angina. The doctor doing the test will watch the wave forms in your ECG as you keep going. You'll be able to stop if the exercise you're being asked to do triggers chest pain. A positive exercise ECG is one when there are significant changes in the wave forms on the ECG during the exercise.

If you've got heart disease, your doctor's going to recommend you take a low dose of aspirin every day. Look at IDEA 17, *Aspirin – the truth*, to understand more about the rationale for this.

Try another idea...

A coronary angiography can confirm the diagnosis of angina. This is done in an X-ray room. A long plastic tube is fed into the artery in your groin, then threaded through your blood vessels and into position in your heart. Dye sent through the catheter shows on a screen so the doctors can see the state of your arteries. The test will let the doctors be sure of your diagnosis and know whether you'd be better off having some sort of heart surgery. Finally, an expensive adenosine stress cardiac MRI scan can look into the coronary arteries in more detail when there's any doubt.

There are two main surgical techniques for people with angina, when medication is not relieving their angina symptoms, or when angina is life-threatening. These are coronary artery bypass surgery and coronary angioplasty: both are to enable more blood to flow through the arteries in your heart.

'A little knowledge can indeed be dangerous but I consider that no knowledge is even more dangerous.'
CHRISTIAAN BARNARD, the first heart transplant surgeon

Defining idea...

How did it go?

Q My dad thought he had indigestion for years. But now he's had some proper tests, it looks as if he's been suffering from angina all the time. Is that common?

A *It can be, yes. Sometimes people think their pain is indigestion because it gets worse when they move about or take exercise after a heavy meal. But if they ignore it, the next thing they know they've had a heart attack. Having an exercise ECG or stress test should detect if the pain is really angina.*

Q I've just been told I've got angina and I've been given loads of drugs. But what can I do for myself?

A *Well, there's lots. Basically you need to reduce your risks of making your heart disease worse so get any risks under control as best you can. If you've got high blood pressure, take medication to get it down, say to 140/85 mmHg or below. If your cholesterol level is high, take a statin drug to lower it. If you've got diabetes, find therapy that gives you tight control so your blood sugar is as near normal levels as possible all day long. Stop smoking if you're a smoker, get your weight down if you're obese, become more active if you're lazy, eat more fruit and vegetables as well as fish (especially oily fish). Ditch stress in your job – either calm down or find another one. Is it too early to retire? You'd have masses more time for walking then...*

34

It's not a life sentence

There are risks with heart surgery, of course there are. But it's more risky to stick your head in the sand and ignore your cardiologist's advice.

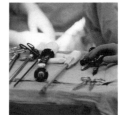

Cardiothoracic surgeons are the stars of the theatre, with anaesthetists, technicians, radiographers and nurses in supporting roles. So it shouldn't be curtains for you.

BEFORE

It's a shock knowing that you're going to go under the knife, and on your heart, too – it can't be happening. But the doctors wouldn't be doing it if there was any other choice for you to be able to live a long life and be as healthy as possible. If you've got angina that isn't being helped much by drugs, they'll probably carry out a coronary angiogram. This will show where your arteries are narrowed and just how narrow they are: it will also find out if any surgery is called for that can control your angina symptoms more effectively and maybe prolong your life.

Before surgery give yourself the best chance. Stop smoking. Get as fit as possible. Lose weight if you're carrying too much fat around. Get a dentist to check that your teeth and gums are healthy and won't be a source of infection after your surgery.

Here's an idea for you... **You've got to have good and unbiased information about the options for heart surgery. Then you can make an informed choice about whether to put up with your symptoms for longer and let your heart come under more strain, or put your trust in the surgeons and go for it. You'll be surprised to learn how low the risks of dying are, even for such major types of surgery. So go to websites such as www.bhf.org.uk or www.americanheart.org to get their fact files and read all about it.**

DURING

Coronary angioplasty is a case of pass the balloon – passing an inflatable balloon from your arm or groin to an artery in your heart. Then, whoosh, pumping up the balloon so that any fatty deposits are squashed flat against the walls of the artery, so the blood flows easily through and your angina disappears. A tube of stainless steel mesh is left behind to hold your artery open and stop it getting blocked again – and that's it.

Then there's a coronary artery bypass. Fixing a blood vessel between your aorta, the main artery leaving your heart, to a point beyond where the blockage is will really improve the blood flow to your heart and relieve you of your angina. The surgeon really works hard for this one. You'll usually be linked up to an artificial heart–lung machine and your scar will be a real showpiece afterwards – right down the length of your breastbone.

You might need work done on your heart valves. There are four valves in your heart, which ensure that your blood flows round on a one-way track: and just like the roads, travelling the wrong way on a one-way system will eventually result in an accident. So if one of your valves is leaky or stiff you'll have problems as the flow of blood will be obstructed. Like a car mechanic, the surgeon's got a choice – leave it alone, repair it or replace it.

AFTER

You'll soon be up and about again, if everything's gone well, and that will help you recover as quickly as possible. Gradually do more activity and exercise once you're home again. You should join in any cardiac rehabilitation programme to build up your fitness and strength. Soon you'll be able to have sex again, and drink alcohol, but don't go back to any of your bad old ways with smoking and drinking and overeating. You'll get better much quicker if you're positive and happy, so try to ban the blues. Stay active, keep your cholesterol down and don't let a particle of tobacco touch your lips. Stay good.

If you're a smoker you really do need to become an ex-smoker, and soon. You'll find help at IDEA 38, *Ready, steady, nearly go*, and IDEA 39, *Quit!*

Try another idea...

PACEMAKERS

One final note. If you've had a pacemaker fitted for your heart block or your irregular heart rhythm, it will have two parts: the power supply or battery and the electronic circuit. It generates electrical impulses that get your heart to contract and produce a beat. The pacemaker is programmed to send electrical impulses to your heart at a rate that suits you; if it senses that your heart rhythm's too slow, for example, it delivers pacing impulses. After a week or so you'll be driving a car again, playing sport and going about life as normal. A pacemaker lasts about six to ten years before needing to be replaced.

'It takes courage to push things forward.'
MO MOWLAM, UK politician

Defining idea...

How did
it go?

Q **If I have a pacemaker fitted will I still be able to use my microwave and my hairdryer?**

A *You can use well-maintained shavers, hairdryers and microwaves just as normal. You'll always have to be careful not to get too close to electromagnetic fields, though, such as at airport security. Just keep walking through any metal detector security systems in shops or libraries. Hold your mobile phone to the ear furthest away from your pacemaker and don't leave it on in a pocket directly over your pacemaker.*

Q **I had surgery on a heart valve five years ago and am still having to take warfarin tablets to thin my blood. Do I really still have to take it, as the regular blood testing's a real nuisance and I'm fine now?**

A *Yes, you must keep taking the tablets, otherwise you risk a clot forming round your heart valve, and that could cause a heart attack or stroke. Then you'd regret that you hadn't bothered with the blood tests every six to eight weeks or so; this really is a case of better safe than sorry.*

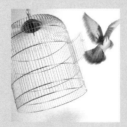

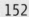

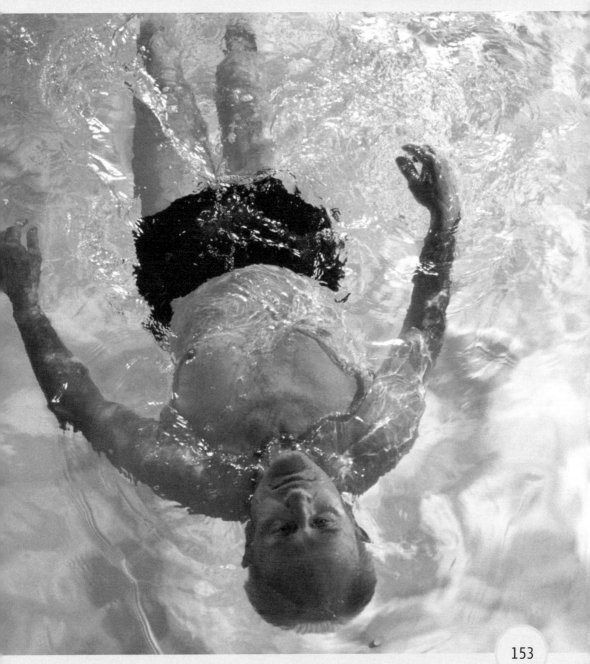

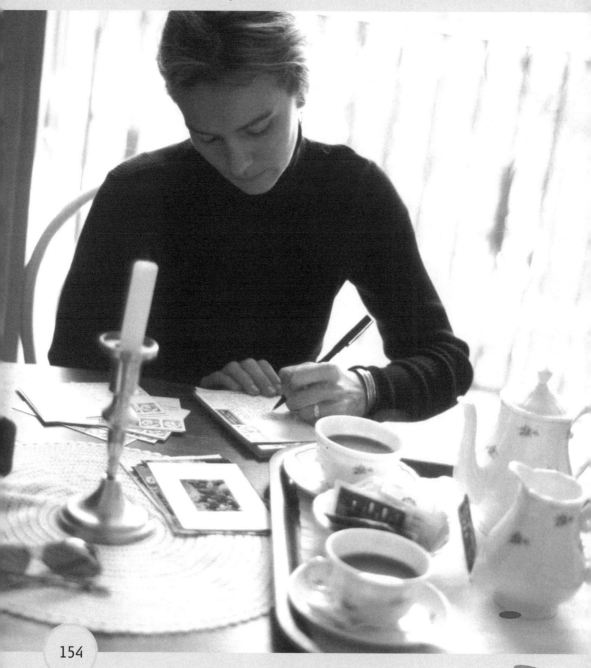

35

At home with the new you

They say charity begins at home. So what's better than being charitable to yourself? Give yourself a fresh start and get rid of your souvenirs from the bad old days.

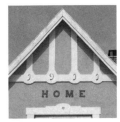

You've turned over a new leaf. Now you want your house to reflect your healthy, changed way of life, so that you're constantly reminded of your good intentions. Your whole house needs a makeover.

There's no smoke in your house, now, except for what comes from the logs on your open fire. So there's no need for ashtrays, then, as you'll be asking visitors to smoke outside from now on. Get rid of any mugs you associate with lighting up in the morning. Replace them with differently coloured mugs, or cups and saucers. Reinforce your vision of a smoke-free life. Drink your coffee or tea in another room or sit at a different seat at the kitchen table from where you used to sit puffing away on your ciggies. Physically move yourself to mirror your different frame of mind as you nurture new habits. Eat your breakfast and other meals where you accept that smoking is forbidden, and don't eat at the kitchen table if you used to routinely smoke there with a meal.

Here's an idea for you...

Redesign your home so that you have some space for exercise – whether that's in the corner of the living room, your bedroom, in the garage or even in the garden. Buy a static bike so you can get busy for chunks of ten minutes at a time, either fitted in when you're at home as a dedicated exercise session or while chatting to the others or watching TV. Equipment for step-ups doesn't take much room; a rowing machine could live in the spare room, so long as you remember to use it. A trampoline in the garden can be for you as well as the kids, so long as it's big enough. Fixing a netball basket on an external wall for shooting goals, or arranging croquet hoops around the lawn, should get you out and practising with your kids or partner.

Redecorate and buy new curtains to get rid of any horrible, stale old smoky smells and stains: once you've stopped, you'll really notice the smell, I promise. Go for a bright and cheerful colour scheme that raises your spirits. Hang pictures of you and your family doing activities that you have obviously enjoyed to encourage you to repeat your experience: climbing mountains, going camping or on cycling holidays together, perhaps.

It might even be worth moving house. Living in the countryside, you will have loads of opportunities to go for a walk or bike ride without needing to set off in a car first. You could move to a small village or town where you get drawn easily into community life and develop new friends. No one will know your old self, and expect you to smoke or drink if they're the habits you're trying to stamp out. Make walkers welcome in your house – with boot racks ready at the door, or a bench and chairs outside in the garden to cluster around. On a less extreme level, if there's any evidence of your bad old way of life then now's the time to do some furniture removal. If you can't hide the evidence of cigarette burns or chocolate stains on something, then its time has come: take it to the tip.

Your newly active way of life may mean that you suffer an aching neck and back for a while until you're truly fit, so you'll want good support from your chairs and bed. Avoid slumping in a sagging armchair, and your bed's got to be firm and give you good support now you've an active life. An over-soft or ancient mattress is no good, so change the mattress if it needs it. Think about buying a better sprung bed or one with a wooden base. Try various beds in the shop to discover just what suits you and your back. You won't want a bad back to stop you from carrying out your new resolution to do regular exercise.

And, finally, don't be so house-proud that there's no room for a dog. After all, a dog could save your life by walking *you* each day. So put up with the doggy footprints padded through your house...

Check out IDEA 1, *Appearances aren't always deceptive*, and fix up plenty of mirrors – they should encourage you to maintain your healthy lifestyle habits.

Try another idea...

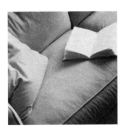

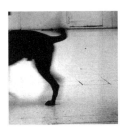

'Home is where the heart is.'
British proverb

Defining idea...

157

How did it go?

Q My flat's in the middle of a busy town. Do you think it would be good to jog a couple of miles or so every morning as part of my new life?

A   *You should avoid air pollution if at all possible. People living close to a main road have twice the chance of dying of heart disease. Maybe this is the time you should consider the health benefits of moving house to a less polluted area? Or exercise indoors – you could call in at the gym on the way to work, or get up at 5 a.m. and jog before there's any traffic about. Is there a nearby park?*

Q My mates have gone feng-shui mad. Is it a lot of hype or could it get me into a more healthy state?

A   *Well, feng shui can use the positive energy of your home environment to boost your good health. The yin and yang energies of your personal space are in a constant state of flux. Creating a yin and yang balance with harmonised levels of light and shade will help you. Fresh flowers, water features, happy family portraits are all part of the picture, and they've got to be pleasant to have about, whether you think feng shui works or not.*

36

Pet theories

Having a pet makes you less prone to heart disease, reduces your stress levels, makes you take exercise you otherwise wouldn't and generally leads you to your healthier life.

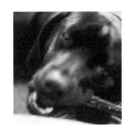

You know you should prevent fur from blocking up your arteries. But fur, as sported by your faithful little pet, can get you out and about and in good form.

A loving home life gladdens your heart and boosts your well-being. Having a cat or dog to come home to means there's always someone pleased to see you, bounding up to greet you after a hard day's work. You won't be lonely with a pet like that and they don't moan or answer back. If you invest attention and love in them, they regard you as being the centre of their world.

Having a pet can raise your spirits, provide you with love and regular exercise – a great trio for your heart. You make resolutions to exercise regularly. But it's hard to do it for yourself when it's cold and wet or you're ultra-tired or just too busy. But if you've got a dog, and it hasn't had its walk that day, then all it takes to get you out

Here's an idea for you... **If you don't fancy being stuck with having to look after and exercise a dog or other pet on a regular basis, you could consider house-sitting as an occasional job. Some owners get so attached to their pets that they pay well to have someone else in their house when they're away so as not to put their pet in kennels. You get to exercise a dog for a week or two when it suits you; it doesn't become a burden and you get paid for doing it. You could get a job at a kennels, of course, exercising the inmates. Homes for abandoned dogs are often looking for volunteer walkers, too.**

there exercising is their soulful, begging eyes: off you go. And you're rewarded by their hysterical excitement, too. If your dog is a twice-a-day walker, then that's before you go off to work and again when you come home. You'll soon do all the walking you're supposed to that way, and you'll extend your social circle by getting to know other dog owners. You might take your pet along while you exercise for company, or even for protection from muggers, running alongside you as you jog or cycle away. If you have the right sort of job, you could take it with you – perhaps while you deliver letters or read meters, for example. Additionally, racing or showing your pet is an absorbing hobby, one that will give you some excitement and challenge and, depending on the type of animal and show, plenty of exercise. Training a collie and practising manoeuvres will have you running further than a marathon every week.

Going up the size scale, keeping a horse will give you a different kind of regular exercise, unless you pay others to train and ride it for racing and other track competitions. Dreaming of riding with the wind in your face, being at one with your animal, will keep you going through gruelling days at work, too.

But a pet can bring you benefits other than exercise, too. Stroking a cat, for example, can help you relax, and caring for an animal can help you climb out of a low mental state. Your pet will give you something else to think about. You can chat to your pet budgie or rat and tell them your problems at the end of the day. Get rid of your angst and relieve your stress; discuss your options with them. They'll listen without interrupting. Just talking out loud will help you think things through – you'll feel all the better for it (and it doesn't mean you're going mad – just the opposite. Much better not to bottle things up).

Finally, you'll be more inclined to trim the fat off food or cut down what you eat, if you give what's left over to your dog or pet rat or whatever, rather than chuck it in the bin. So your pet will, indirectly, even encourage you to eat more healthily.

Pets are especially good feng shui in homes left empty during the day. Look at IDEA 35, *At home with the new you*, for other ways of changing your house.

Try another idea...

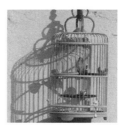

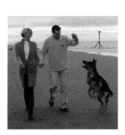

'Animals are such agreeable friends – they ask no questions, they pass no criticisms.'
GEORGE ELIOT

Defining idea...

How did
it go?

Q **Has the pet got to be a four-legged animal or would a snake or tarantula fit the bill?**

A *A snake or spider might give other people a heart attack when they catch sight of them, but if you like them, they'll distract you from the daily grind and make you happy – and that's good for your heart.*

Q **I live in a very small flat, so although I'd love a big dog like a labrador, I think only a chihuahua would fit in. Would a little dog like that help my heart?**

A *Well, you'd be able to stroke a chihuahua more easily than a labrador; it would sit happily on your lap for hours on end. However, it wouldn't want to walk miles with you and you'd probably end up carrying it on country walks... but they're not heavy, so that will still be good for your heart.*

Q **Are there any disadvantages to having pets, as far as my heart's concerned?**

A *If you suffer from asthma you might be allergic to fur, and your worsening asthma might put more strain on your heart. Dogs and cats and other animals generally have quite short lifespans compared to us, so every so often you'll have to cope with their death, but you may well cut short your grieving by getting your next pet, of course. Many people do.*

37

Have fun

Life can't be all fun – but most of it can. So be greedy for fun.

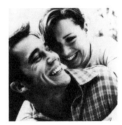

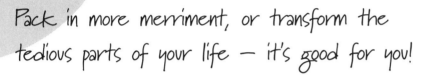
Pack in more merriment, or transform the tedious parts of your life — it's good for you!

You are what you do. Get a balanced diet of activities in your life: you have your basic chores and work to get through so make them count towards your fun index. Then make sure there's enough time for you to enjoy yourself. Here are some ideas.

FUN AT WORK

- Work within limits. As far as you can, limit your working hours to what's reasonable. Don't cheat by reclassifying some aspect of your work as a hobby, so you can work on it at night and through the weekends. And don't take work away on holiday – no laptop, no mobile phone, so work contacts cannot reach you: and no sneaking off to access emails sent to your work address.

- Make time for fun. Rediscover jokes if you've lost touch with them. Get in an email network where jokes are circulated. They lighten the daily chore of processing your emails and get you laughing spontaneously, though any work colleagues not sharing your jokes and hearing you laugh might wonder if you were losing it... Suggest joke competitions for team days at work – organise

Here's an idea for you...

You're a kid at heart. So if you've got young children or maybe grandchildren, actively enjoy their company. Live in the present with them, don't hanker after the long list of jobs you've set yourself or hope that another adult will rescue you soon. Laugh with them at the simple but ridiculous things they find funny. You'll feel better for it. Sit on the floor and play their games, race along yanking a kite, roll around in play fights or accept their simple hugs – all good fun that can only benefit your heart.

prizes for the best joke, the worst joke teller, the most awful pun, etc. That'll lighten the mood and get a team bonding quicker than any consultant facilitator can manage.

■ The fun index at some workplaces can be quite low, so up the level. Organise some team outings to the cinema, or maybe bowling, so everyone can join in. Be imaginative and find ways to have fun together that are not at anyone's expense. Even in the most dire workplaces it's fun that gets you through: medics are notorious for their gruesome sense of humour, but what else can you do when you're coping with death or dying? Even the grimmest office can be improved.

GROWN-UP FUN

■ Everyone needs time for adult fun. That's not necessarily tied up with sex or drinking, though it could be if that's your thing (and you're not drinking to excess, of course). It's preserving time when you can do what you want to do, do what makes you happy. And if you're happy, your heart

Defining idea...

'*Happiness writes white; it does not show up on the page.*'
HENRY DE MONTHERLANT, French essayist

will be happy. So work out how much time you can afford, or need, to stay sane and cope with the pressures upon you for the rest of your week. Maybe it's three evenings

Have some fun with your pet. Check out IDEA 36, *Pet theories*, for more.

Try another idea...

a week or the equivalent spread over the weekend. So you can exercise at the gym, go for a run, dine out with friends without feeling guilty. You'll probably work more effectively for it, so it's a win–win situation all round. Don't feel guilty that you're spending time on yourself, doing what you want to do, enjoying yourself and having fun.

- Try something new. You could try developing a new hobby or skill at least once a year: do something you've always meant to do but not got round to. Timetable it into your time out, or make an arrangement or pay a deposit or do something concrete that commits you to getting on with it. What about learning the flute, doing some art and craft, or brushing up on your French or Italian, for instance?

- Browse in a book or music store. Select something different you've never heard of or sampled before. Extend your horizons. Find out what amuses and pleases you. The music itself could be a calming influence on your heart as well as interesting you and making you come alive – which is also good for your heart. Reading could transport you from your everyday cares and destress you – another healthy boost for your heart.

Finally, take time to reflect on what your life's about. Hopefully you'll realise there's no point in being too serious. No one knows the answer to the major philosophical questions, so you might as well have fun and feel good while you wait for the mysteries of life to be revealed.

'Happy the man, and happy he alone, He who can call today his own; He who secure within, can say "Tomorrow do thy worst, for I have lived today".'
HORACE

Defining idea...

How did it go?

Q **Having fun's all very well, but some people overdo it. How can I stop my stupid colleagues messing about so much that I'm not the one doing the extra work?**

A *They're adults, so let them take the consequences of their own actions. Don't cover for them; they'll continue to mess about while you're prepared to do their work. And do try to lighten up a bit, or the stress you're bringing on yourself will have dire consequences...*

Q **Is all fun good for you, whatever the source? Would you include bungy jumping or hang-gliding or are they too dangerous?**

A *If you've a bulge in one of your arteries, it could burst when you do that bungy jump and kill or paralyse you with a stroke. Hang-gliding can be dangerous like that, too. It's all a matter of you balancing the risks and benefits to you. Don't get addicted to risk so that anything a bit tamer is no fun for you.*

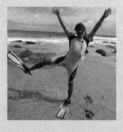 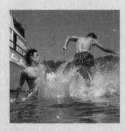 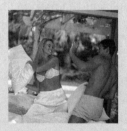

38

Ready, steady, nearly go

Willpower is what you need to develop if you're going to stop smoking. Being quick on the draw is really shooting yourself in the foot.

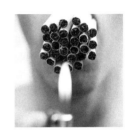

The likelihood of you giving up depends on how well prepared you are...

It also depends on how motivated you are to stop, how addicted you are to nicotine and what support you get. Seven out of ten smokers want to stop, and four out of five wish they'd never started.

HERE'S SOME HELP

- Get ready. Think through what you'll gain from stopping smoking. Divide a page of paper in half and put the benefits of stopping smoking on one side and what you'll lose on the other. Losing your cough, losing the stale smell once you've quit – these count as benefits and not negatives!

- Set the date. D Day. That's Definitely Stop Day. That's *cross my heart and hope to die, I mean it* day. You are going to stop.

- Throw away all the trappings. These are things that have you in the smoking trap: your lighters, those spare boxes of matches, the ashtrays, the hidden

Here's an idea for you...

Stop smoking with others: take a group pledge to quit. Swop phone numbers and all stop smoking on the same day. Then you can email, telephone or text among yourselves to boost each other and keep up your resolve. You might even have some money riding on the result. If you've got no smoking buddy to give up with, then you can arrange a 'textmereminder' service to send you regular text messages to your mobile phone – or leave messages on your landline phone – to remind you not to light up. You can set them to arrive at your most vulnerable times.

packets of cigarettes or any cigars hoarded for a special occasion. Be prepared; scout around and remove anything, absolutely anything, that might tempt you into smoking again.

■ Get a store of distractions for when you're craving a cigarette. Chewing gum will keep your fingers busy unwrapping papers and give your mouth something active to do (besides swearing about quitting). Make sure it's sugar-free gum, or you'll be ruining your teeth. Chop up some raw vegetables or fruit, like carrots or an apple, that you can chomp on. Turn to drink – but the non-alcoholic kind like water, sugar-free drinks or decaffeinated ones. Frequent sips will keep your fingers and mouth occupied. Worry beads could provide finger therapy, too.

■ Tell everyone your plan. Get them on your side at home, at work and in the pub. You need the gang to look out for you, support you in giving up, stop you from having another cigarette – ever again. Unfortunately, there's always one so-called friend – or two, or ten – who is likely to tempt you back to your bad old ways, in order to keep them company. So make it a challenge for them: don't give in, don't be a walkover.

■ Think positive. Yes, yes, yes: you can do it. If you get withdrawal symptoms, that's great, the nicotine's becoming a thing of the past. If your concentration's poor, then fantastic: you're at least focusing on not smoking. If you're craving something to eat, wonderful – you're enjoying food even more.

This is a really difficult thing for people to do; you might need more motivation. So read IDEA 39, *Quit!* to get that extra help. IDEA 52, *You know it...* can help here, too.

Try another idea...

■ Change your routine, especially in the first week which will be the most difficult. Walk to work or cycle, rather than take the bus or train. It'll make you feel better and reinforce your new healthy way of life. Don't go to the places you used to go to smoke or you'll risk slipping into your bad old haze. You could avoid the pub and go to a no-smoking restaurant instead. Keep away from the staff rest room if that's where people congregate to smoke and take a stroll instead, or find another room where you won't be tempted. You're a new person now.

■ Reward yourself: but not with a cigarette! After all, you've been saving all that money you would otherwise have spent on fags, so spend your ciggie money on actual things that you can see – clothes, music, whatever – as a tangible proof of your achievement.

And lastly, do remember the statistics. On average, persistent smokers will die ten years younger than non-smokers. The risk of dying in middle age is three times as great for a smoker – and 33% of non-smokers survive until they're ninety, compared to only 7% of smokers.

'Yes, it hurt; yes, it worked.'
British political slogan

Defining idea...

How did it go?

Q   It's so difficult to stop smoking, I don't think I care any more about trying. Can you suggest something to motivate me?

A   *If you can't stop smoking for your own sake, can you do it for others? By regularly exposing your family or colleagues to your second-hand smoke you're increasing their risk of lung cancer and heart disease by 24%. Babies and children get coughs, wheezing and bronchitis from passive smoking as their lungs are more delicate, and they'll be three times more likely to get lung cancer themselves when they're older. If you're inflicting your smoking on a pregnant woman, then her baby will be smaller – and she'll be more likely to have a stillbirth.*

Q   How much is my asthma likely to improve if I stop smoking?

A   *In brief, a lot. If you stop, your asthma will be more easily controlled as smoking impairs the effectiveness of steroid inhalers that are key for your asthma. And you'll be less likely to be admitted to hospital, too.*

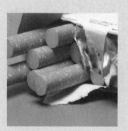

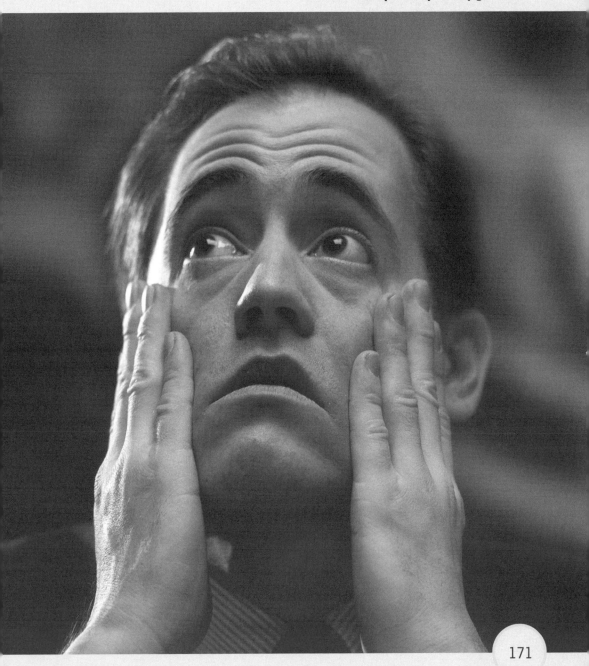

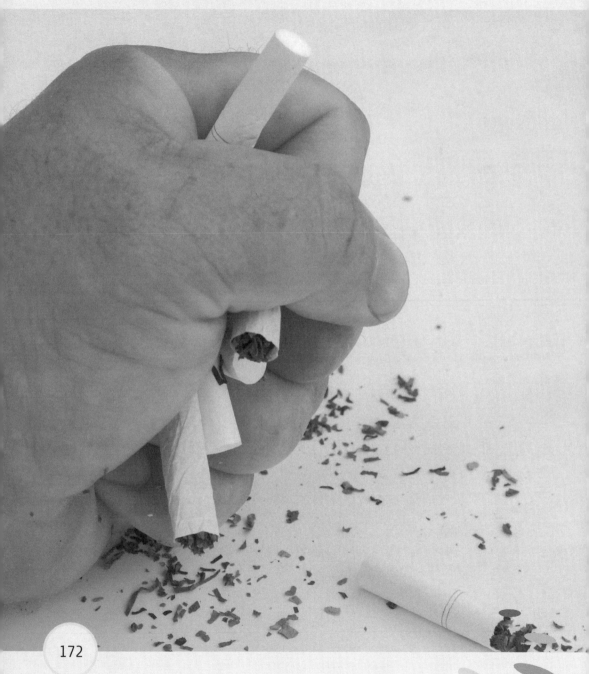

39

Quit!

Smokers quickly get fagged out if they go on a run or do some heavy work. If you've tried to stop, and haven't found the willpower, here are some things to try.

If having a healthy lifestyle gets you lit up, then you'll want to quit while you're ahead. It's hard, though — but people can help.

Just remember: if you've a death wish, then smoking's for you. Of the 4000 or so chemicals in tobacco smoke, at least 60 cause cancer... But if you're a smoker, you know this, so how can you stop?

HERE ARE SOME IDEAS

- You can double your chances of quitting smoking successfully by using nicotine replacement therapies such as patches, lozenges, inhalers or gum. These can reduce your cravings by giving you enough nicotine to ease your withdrawal symptoms. Doctors can prescribe these or you can buy them yourself.

- Another option is taking buproprion under medical supervision. This drug suppresses the nicotine buzz and lessens your withdrawal symptoms. It acts on

Use phototherapy to increase your determination to quit and stop forever. A picture paints a thousand words – and hopefully all of these are 'I must not start smoking again' repeated many times over. Nothing ages your skin, hair and nails faster than smoking. Take a good look at the diseased hearts and lungs of smokers displayed on posters and now even on cigarette packets. Pin them up wherever you are most tempted to start smoking again. You could always take a digital photo of yourself and then alter it so that it looks prematurely aged – wrinkles, thread veins, disgusting teeth – and remember that you might well end up looking like that if you don't stop.

'Change will lead to insight far more than insight will lead to change.'
MILTON ERICHSON, hypnotherapist

your brain, quelling your desire to smoke and easing withdrawal symptoms such as being irritable and restless. It takes a week to kick in, so you might start it and then stop smoking in the second week. The course lasts for two months.

■ There are lots of stop-smoking helplines which provide free advice and information. Cessation clinics or self-help groups could give you the support you need if your willpower isn't enough.

■ Ear acupuncture can be very effective in helping to combat your craving for nicotine, and it will also help to relieve anxiety and stress brought on by withdrawal symptoms when you quit. The usual 'Western' approach is to insert a few fine needles (perhaps three or four) for around twenty minutes or so. With the Chinese approach, needles may be left in for up to an hour. Rotating the needles in the skin keeps re-stimulating the acupuncture point. Different acupuncturists use various techniques; they vary as to the sites of the body, the lengths of time needles are left in and whether they attach small electric currents to the needles (electroacupuncture) or use heated herbs (moxa) to warm the needles. Disposable needles are usually used, as they are reasonably cheap.

Hypnotherapy works well to help some people stop smoking. Look at IDEA 20, *Hypnotherapy – more, more...* for information.

Try another idea...

YOUR RECOVERY TIME

The benefits start as soon as you quit. Just eight hours after your last ciggie, the oxygen levels in your blood return to normal and your risk of having a heart attack starts to fall. After twenty-four hours the carbon monoxide leaves your body and your lungs start to clear out mucous and other debris. By seventy-two hours, your taste and smell have improved, your breathing is already easier and you've more energy. Your clot risk plunges only fourteen days after stopping smoking. Three months later your circulation has improved and exercise is easier. After a year, your risk of having a heart attack has dropped to about half that of a smoker and after ten years, your risk of lung cancer will have fallen to half that of a smoker. Fifteen years on, and your risk of a heart attack is about the same as that of someone who has never smoked.

'For every thousand 20-year-old smokers it is estimated that one will be murdered, six will die in a road accident and 250 will die in middle age from smoking!'
Imperial Cancer Research Fund and World Health Organisation

Defining idea...

Q   I've succeeded in quitting smoking and I really, really want to stay stopped. Have you any tips on how to stop myself relapsing and having another?

A   *If you've got someone who takes a real interest in you stopping, then you won't want to let them down. That could be a doctor or nurse, your partner, a parent, your child or best friend. Some people say that listening to repeated recorded messages telling them to stop smoking, in a quiet room with no distractions, can help reinforce their determination – so it might be worth trying. If you do slip up and have one, don't think all is lost and start off smoking again: keep a positive mindset. Don't give up on giving up.*

Q   I'm tempted to try quitting using buproprion. Are there any side effects?

A   *Yes. You might experience insomnia, a dry mouth, anxiety, headaches and nausea, but the side effects of carrying on smoking if you don't try it might be worse than anything you'd get from using the drug. However, anyone with epilepsy or with some severe mental health problems, women who are pregnant or breast feeding shouldn't take it.*

Q   How can using patches be good for you when they're just giving you extra nicotine?

A   *Your main target is to stop smoking, and an extra few weeks of nicotine from the patches is inconsequential in the long term. Soon you'll be reducing the strength of the patches and gradually tailing them off, and then you'll be looking at a nicotine-free life.*

40

Travel assurance

Get off to a flying start on your holiday or business trip. You want to enjoy your time away, not worry about your health, so prepare well and you'll ensure trouble-free travel.

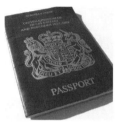

There's a lot you can do to stay healthy on your trip whether you've a history of heart disease, or a perfectly normal heart and circulation that you want to stay that way.

Here are a few tips to help you on your journey.

- Take enough medicines to last your whole holiday, with some spare medication for luck – in case you're delayed on your return home, or have some sort of mishap with your tablets. If your medication is critical, like for treating diabetes, carry some in your hand luggage as well as in your main suitcase. Keep a record of what you're taking, and keep it separate from your drugs. Use their generic rather than trade names, so that they are recognisable worldwide. Then you'll be able to replace them fairly easily if your medication is stolen or your baggage goes missing.

Here's an idea for you... **Wear a pair of below-the-knee socks to prevent a blood clot forming in the deep veins of your calves if you're going on a long-haul flight. You're more likely to have trouble on flights lasting five hours or more, or covering a distance of 3000 miles or further. It could also be a car, coach or train journey lasting the same length of time without a break. You can buy elastic compression socks or stockings from pharmacies and supermarkets. Class 1 compression gives the recommended 14–17 mmHg pressure.**

- Don't rush about at the last minute toting heavy suitcases. All that rushing and stress could put your blood pressure up. Plan your travel carefully and anticipate any blips, so there are no last minute panics.

- If you've got a pacemaker fitted, you can still fly but let airport security know so you don't get too close to any electromagnetic field that interferes with it. If you've had a recent heart attack you'll need to take advice about whether you are fit to fly; check with your insurance company what cover you've got. In general, a heart attack or recent surgery in the previous ten days will require clearance from an airline's medical adviser before you travel.

- Come clean about your health problems when taking out holiday insurance, even if you're in good health when booking. Otherwise, if you have related problems while on holiday, your insurance policy may be void. You'll need good cover if you're going far afield where there are no reciprocal health service arrangements with the country you're visiting, so shop around for insurance companies with client-friendly policies for people with heart disease. Europeans travelling in the European Union need an E111 form completed and stamped. The E111 arrangements don't cover repatriation, though. So go for minimum medical insurance cover in the 3 million euros bracket for medical, surgical and dental costs – they soon add up if you need a difficult repatriation home. Carry proof of insurance with you at all times.

One thing that worries people is the risk of a blood clot forming. So here's how to cut the risks. Now, some individuals are more at risk of a clot forming in their blood vessels or heart anyway, even if they weren't going to travel. These are people who don't move about much –

Look at IDEA 17, *Aspirin – the truth*, for a reminder on how taking a low dose of aspirin before you board the aeroplane for a long-haul flight can help.

Try another idea...

they may have a plaster cast on their leg or be paralysed in some way; be women who are pregnant, on HRT or the contraceptive pill; or be obese people or those with cancer. People who've had a thrombosis in the past are more likely to have one again.

Everyone can minimise their chances of a clot forming while they're travelling by plane, train or car via some simple measures. During the trip, bend and straighten your legs, feet and toes every half hour. Take occasional short walks if you can – down the aisle of the plane or train, or at service stations if you're travelling by car. Drink plenty of water and don't drink too much alcohol so you don't get dehydrated – or comatose! Avoid taking sleeping tablets, as you might sleep slumped, without moving. If you're at risk of a clot then wear elastic stockings.

Take some exercise before you fly and after you arrive at your destination. You can go walking, cycling or swimming before you fly out, depending on the time of day – though swimming in a local icy stream at 3 a.m. or being arrested for breaking into the local pool does not sound a good way to start your holiday…

'To travel hopefully is a better thing than to arrive.'
ROBERT LOUIS STEVENSON

Defining idea...

How did it go?

Q **My angina's pretty stable and I feel well. I've got to go on a business trip to Canada soon and it's likely to be quite stressful as a lot depends on our sales there. What should I do if my angina gets worse while I'm away?**

A *Carry a copy of your latest electrocardiogram (ECG) with you, and a list of your medication and brief personal medical details of your condition. Then, if you have to see a doctor, they can decide if any changes on your ECG are something different or just old news. Include contact numbers for physicians and relatives at home in your wallet.*

Q **My sister has had a deep vein thrombosis (DVT) in the past and is nervous of flying with us on holiday this year. Is there anything else she can do to be safe?**

A *Travellers who've had a DVT before like your sister, or who've got several risk factors, can be given a single injection of the blood-thinning drug heparin under their skin two or three hours before they fly. This injection will thin the blood almost immediately for up to twelve hours. Your sister should ask her doctor how to arrange this for both outward and return travel.*

41

Break away

Break away from the office and the daily hassles. Put your heart into having a great holiday with lots of activity.

Look upon your holiday as an opportunity to undo the bad effects of your everyday life, and boost your energy stores so you come home revitalised.

There are lots of things to remember to make your holiday a holiday for your heart, too.

Let's start with luggage. Choose your suitcases carefully, so that when full they're not too heavy. Even with the ones with wheels, you'll still have to lift your bags sometimes, which could be a strain for you. Pack your stuff in two small suitcases rather than one big, heavy one. Don't get distracted by the children squabbling or time pressures – concentrate on lifting your cases in a way that avoids too much effort for your heart, or straining your back. Take plenty of loose change for tipping porters; they want to carry your cases and you're on holiday and want to take it easy: it's a win–win situation.

181

Here's an idea for you...

Opt for an all-inclusive holiday. You thought 'all inclusive' meant all you can eat and drink packed into a stay at a hotel, didn't you? Well, try thinking of all inclusive as meaning as much exercise and activity as you can manage to fit in, instead – with the food and drink there just to give you the energy to do your activities.

It might be tempting to take a holiday from your diet too, but it's a case of feast your eyes rather than your stomach and sticking it out for the sake of your healthy heart. Your meals can still be delicious. Take a sugar substitute with you, go for low-fat options, avoid creamy deserts and have lots of salads and low-calorie drinks. If you're browsing the buffet in a hotel, then do your best to fill up your plate with lots of salad, vegetables, fish and fruit. Have a squeeze of lemon juice instead of a dollop of mayonnaise. And try and make an alcoholic drink last for ages.

You could always book a really healthy holiday. If you've got any bad habits – smoking, drinking heavily, being inactive, overeating – then make up your mind to change your behaviour and change it forever. You've probably felt guilty about your bad habit(s) for some time and made several resolutions to change, and then relapsed. What better way to learn more about how you must change, and see the benefits of a healthy lifestyle, than booking in at a health farm? Let your stay there be the first day of the rest of your life: eat a healthy diet, take regular and varied exercise, relax and enjoy yourself, don't smoke and just drink alcohol in moderation. Perhaps making all those changes at once is asking a bit much, but start somewhere and improve your lifestyle in a staged way. If actually staying at a health farm is out of your price range, you could just go for the day out of season when there's a special offer.

If you're staying somewhere there's a gym, then use it. Book in for a session with a personal trainer. Find out what possible activities you could do, so you can experiment with new approaches. Swop health tips with others there, and watch how they use the gym equipment. Learn from them and try their ways yourself.

Check out IDEA 6, *Kick-start your exercise*, for more on physical activity.

Try another idea...

If you're not as active at home as you should be, then try and incorporate physical activity of the right kind into your holiday, or health farm break. That will be great for your heart. If you do a sport that's new to you or one for which you're out of practice, take it easy at first. Pace yourself and build up the time you spend on it over successive days; you don't always realise that you've overdone things until you wake up, stiff and in pain, the following day.

Holidays don't have to be solely about exercise, though. Your holiday should be a happy change from your routine, when you can do things you don't normally have enough time to try; these could be activities like painting or creative writing, or you could simply take time to enjoy the fresh air and the countryside or garden flowers while you're away – to raise your spirits.

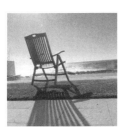

'What an odd thing tourism is. You fly off to a strange land, eagerly abandoning all the comforts of home, and then expend vast quantities of time and money in a largely futile attempt to recapture the comforts that you wouldn't have lost if you hadn't left home in the first place.'
BILL BRYSON, travel writer

Defining idea...

183

How did
it go?

Q I'd love to go on an all-inclusive or long-haul holiday, or trot off to a health spa, but they're not in my price bracket. Can you give me some affordable tips?

A   *Just staying at home and walking and cycling round to discover what your neighbourhood offers could make a great break. You can't get cheaper than that. Local leisure centre gyms are often very cheap to use, too. Volunteering for something like a regeneration project will give you a cheap and active holiday, and lots of opportunities to meet new friends. You'll come back worn out, but fitter than when you went.*

Q Physical activity? I'm so worn out from work all I want to do is to collapse on a sun lounger when I'm on holiday. What hope is there for me?

A   *After you've rested for a couple of days, do get some exercise incorporated into your day. It can be gentle: a swim before breakfast, a walk along the beach to the next resort. Check out the hotel gym. After dinner, get up and go for a walk – that'll aid your digestion, as well.*

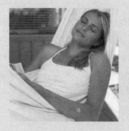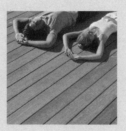

42

Don't kid yourself

Look after your kids and they'll look after you – so it's a good investment to bring them up in a healthy way.

As children are so impressionable, everyone involved in their lives needs to give them consistently healthy messages. And it's never too early to start.

BEFORE BIRTH, THEN PRE-SCHOOL

What happens in pregnancy will have repercussions: smoking or drinking too much alcohol, or flooding them with fat and carbohydrates so they're on the chubby side themselves – even before they're born. Once they are born, let everyone know you're going to bring them up in a healthy way, so the kind of presents people will give can reflect that. A pram or baby carrier, that will let you roam round the countryside, rather than a fashion accessory, for shopping; maybe a food processor for preparing home-cooked baby meals.

Your children may not be able to read or write but they'll recognise the food and drink you favour. Sugary sweets and fizzy drinks aren't worth their fervent hugs and thanks; give them non-edible rewards for good behaviour, like stars on a reward

Here's an idea for you... **Develop a mutual love of a shared activity with your kids so you go rock climbing or sailing together eagerly, and keep each other participating even when you're tired and it's all a lot of effort. You'll have lots more in common, then, and that'll keep you together as a family even in the potentially dangerous teenage years, when your kids might drift over to unhealthy influences.**

chart, your time for doing activities, new crayons or similar arty things. And keep a watch on their weight to height ratio for their age. You may have got so used to everyone being overweight that you need to relearn what a normal weight looks like.

Now, don't let them get used to watching too much TV. OK, you're not perfect and television and videos are good distractions for kids from time to time when your energy levels or patience are low. If they do watch something which features people with bad lifestyle habits on it, explain why what they are doing is bad, especially if they're the stars of the show. But time your kids spend sitting in front of the TV is time they could have been running around instead. Enrol them in an activity club – dancing or sport of some kind – and convince them that sport and exercise are good if you can: that mantra has got to stick with them for life.

If you have a bad habit like smoking cigarettes or illicit drugs, then hide it from the children, though you should try to stop for their sakes, if not your own. Don't let them see you as the role model they're going to emulate unconsciously when they grow up.

SCHOOLDAYS ONWARDS

Keep schooling them in healthy ways. Read up on how to instil effective health messages and see what the experts think. As they get older, you've got to become cleverer at manipulating them into leading healthy lives, seemingly by their own choice and not because you're nagging them continually.

The school should be on your side. See what you can do to reinforce healthy messages put out at school in projects or at school events. Encourage them to join in after-school clubs that get them outside, playing games. They need an hour of moderate physical activity seven days a week if possible – got to get them into those good habits...

Hopefully, by now they'll have come to love your home cooking and the low-fat, healthy balanced meals you dish out. Make sure there are healthy options at times like Halloween; don't just go for treacle toffee or toffee apples, but other fruity alternatives too, such as strawberries coated in chocolate or grapes, cherries and orange segments arranged on cocktail sticks like a fruity kebab. Birthday parties could focus more on activities, like having a swimming party with healthy snacks and fruit, rather than a big fuss round a birthday tea. And you could play pass the parcel so that the final present unwrapped is something to do instead of something to eat.

It's even more important for children to get used to food without salt than it is for adults. Check up on IDEA 14, Salt away.

Try another idea...

'Children have never been very good at listening to their elders, but they have never failed to imitate them. They must, they have no other models.'
JAMES BALDWIN, author

Defining idea...

Q **I have long working hours and little time or energy. What can I do to educate my kids to make healthy choices about how they behave?**

A *Could their grandparents step in when you're not around to take them out, be role models or give them sensible advice? Go for family holidays on the move, rather than beach squatting or touring. Fine, you're worn out from work and want to flake out. But go somewhere you can have a couple of days recuperating while the kids join in organised activities or do their own thing, and where once you've recovered there are lots of opportunities for family play: swimming, racket sports, skating, the playground – things like that.*

Q **Our kids are computer and TV addicts. They'd rather fiddle with their games than play football. Any way we can get them moving?**

A *You're adults, aren't you? Stronger and cleverer than your kids. You could do heavy stuff like banning computer games alternate months so they get used to life without them, or just sell the games and use the money to buy bikes. Then you could always make sure the TV reception's so poor that it's not worth watching! Keep calling on them to help you in the garden or with your pets, or simply organise some really attention-grabbing alternative activities, so they want to join in real life rather than play make-believe on screen.*

43

Dressing the part

You can still look stunning when you're out there running. But you can't walk or run any distance unless you're comfortable, so make sure you wear the right gear.

Or maybe dressing down suits you better — it doesn't take long to throw on a tracksuit, no make-up, no hairstyling — just up and off, and get your heart pumping.

You've got to dress for success when playing sports. You want to wear clothes you feel comfortable in so you can move freely, and good sports shoes that let you walk or run for miles and miles without getting callouses or blisters. And walking or running are such great exercises for your heart: you need to do everything you can to be able to do them. Go for robust, well-fitting shoes or flat-soled walking sandals that can be strapped on tightly. And don't let bad weather keep you indoors. You can't put maintaining the health of your heart on hold just because it's cold or wet. Buy yourself some good outside gear so the only dampness you'll feel will be healthy sweat – and not even that, if you can believe the ads for expensive jackets made of material which 'lets your body breathe and wicks away sweat'.

Here's an idea for you... **Wear fashionable clothes. You want to portray a youthful image, don't you? So that means being up to date, though not attracting ridicule by following a too-young look. Your regular exercising, healthy diet and triumph over bad personal habits will mean you glow with health. So do yourself justice and craft a young-looking, modern image too. Others will respond to your youthful image in our increasingly ageist society and that'll help keep up your resolution to stick to healthy routines.**

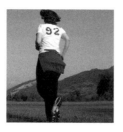

Always remember that you can't run or reach for that low ball if your clothing is too tight. The cheapest solution might be to lose a few kilos so your clothes are baggy, but that might take time... so go for material that stretches without being baggy, even when it's been washed loads of times. And if you do intentionally lose lots of weight, then throw away your old clothes and enjoy your slim frame, wearing close-fitting, but stretchy, things. If you've got to buy lots of replacement clothes, it'll be a great incentive not to relapse and put more weight back on.

Your eyes are important and you should be ready to shield them from the sun when you take all this healthy exercise. Perhaps you fancy yourself with a sun shield, rather than a cap, like professional golfers wear? Maybe a cap is better if you're at all balding: remember it's not just your eyes that need protection from the sun. It may be time to convert to contact lenses rather than glasses for sports that require you to bound about, or use sideways vision. It's never too late to try contact lenses even if you've stuck to glasses all your life; if you last tried them some time ago, you may be surprised at how they've changed.

And finally, celebrate your trophies, don't be shy. You know how good people feel with trophies connected to their achievements stacked around them. Well this kind of idea can work for you too. You could choose kit, or maybe ties or blouses, to reflect your healthy athletic image, or membership of a particular sports club. That keeps reminding you and everyone else of your interest in and commitment to sport and exercise. Reinforcement like that works well.

Go for a jacket or coat with pockets when walking the dog. Look at IDEA 36, *Pet theories*, if you need more convincing that it's worth planning for a pet.

Try another idea...

'Dress up a stick and it does not appear to be a stick.'
English proverb

Defining idea...

Q   My brother's promised to get me running with him. Any advice on what kind of shoes I should wear?

How did it go?

A   *You could get a proper biomechanics assessment of your feet from a podiatrist so you know something about whether you've normal pronation, or are an overpronator (have 'duck feet') or underpronator (that's being pigeon-toed, for the uninitiated). Then you can select running shoes that give you stability, cushion you against the impact of running, or aid your flexibility and motion. If you can't afford that, go to a sports shop and get them to explain the advantages of the various types they stock, try them on carefully and decide what'll suit you. Take your time to get this right.*

Q   **My friend's still upset about her father dying young from a heart attack recently. How can I motivate her to join me in getting fit?**

A   *Is she big on appearances? Could you buy her a T-shirt that supports a national heart charity? Those are getting very smart these days. Then get her to start running and training with you so she could enter a half-marathon or some similar event wearing that T-shirt, perhaps raising money for the charity.*

Q   **My man's got everything. And I mean everything. What surprise present can I buy him to wear which might help get him healthy?**

A   *Does he like high-tech gizmos? Does he have more digital toys than digits already? Well, he'd love one more, surely. How about getting him to wear a global positioning system (GPS) running computer on his wrist? It looks like a watch, but will compute exactly where he is when he's out running or walking, how far he's gone and what speed he moves at, even the number of calories of energy it's taken. It'll keep a record of every exercise session and do a detailed analysis so he can compare what he does on one particular day with another.*

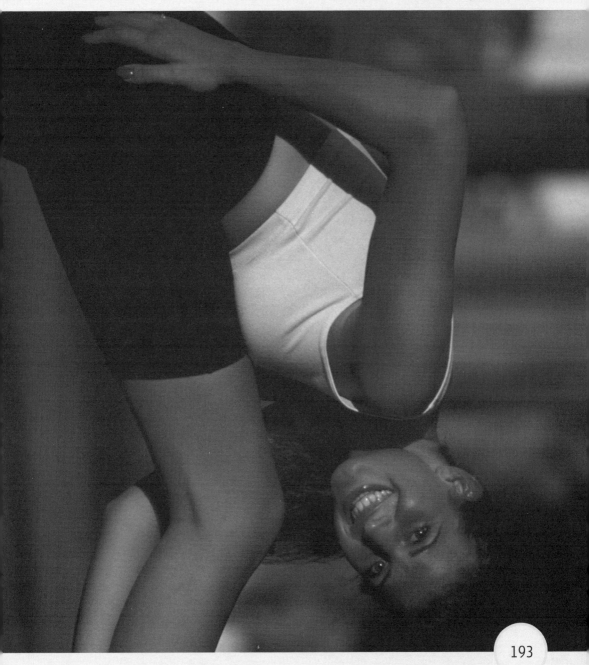

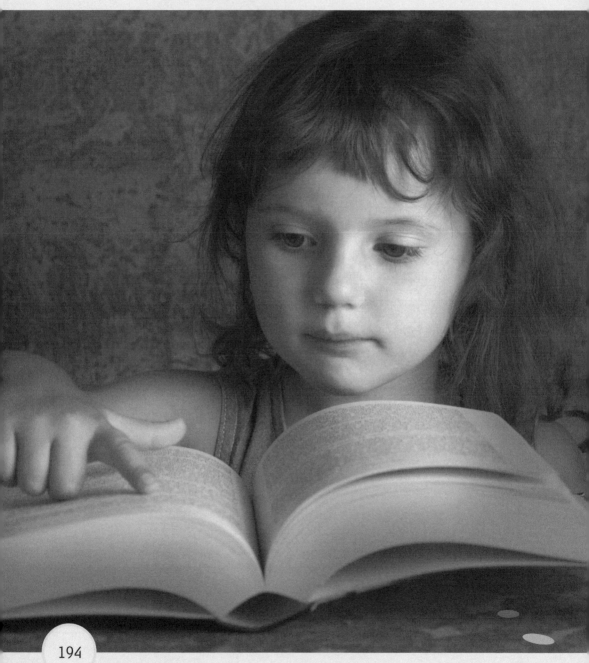

44

A heart-warming read

Don't underestimate the power of the written word. You can use it, and in many different ways, to help you improve the health of your heart.

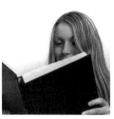

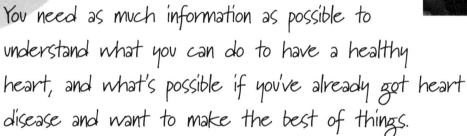

You need as much information as possible to understand what you can do to have a healthy heart, and what's possible if you've already got heart disease and want to make the best of things.

Everywhere you look there are articles and tips about what to do to help your heart stay healthy. Open a magazine at random and, sure enough, there'll be something useful about your health. When you read it, you think you'll remember it, but five minutes later you'll be distracted and forget. So why not start a scrapbook? Cut out or copy those articles from the health columns in newspapers, or from free booklets you pick up at the doctor's or when loitering in supermarket queues. Preserve those healthy tips for your heart. Create sections in your scrapbook, so there's material about good lifestyles, for example, and a focus on anything you're specially interested in, like getting your cholesterol down. Perhaps you could have a section for recipes that look tantalisingly delicious while at the same time being healthy. Put some old pictures of you in your scrapbook, maybe something you're aiming to repeat on the front cover – you much slimmer, you active, and you looking healthy. Include mottoes or sayings you think will motivate you.

Read case studies of success: stories about how people you can identify with beat their addictions to smoking or drinking too much alcohol. How couch potatoes made good. How people became the slimming kings or queens of the year, despite the odds. How they emerged as healthy role models, despite pressures in their lives. Yes, you might prefer to read celebrity stories, but they're difficult to believe and their circumstances are so different from yours that their cases aren't really comparable.

'Reading is to the mind what exercise is to the body.'
RICHARD STEELE, journalist

A word of caution, though. Don't forget that what you collect or snip out may well be biased and not reliable. It may really be a disguised advert – they're often called 'advertorials' in magazines – for a particular product. It may look like a learned piece on a subject – one that just happens to end up strongly recommending that you try a particular food or medicine and almost frightens you into buying it. So keep a note of where you got your scrap of paper or article from, in case you want to follow up the source at a later date.

HERE ARE A FEW MORE IDEAS

■ You could write yourself a personal message on a postcard, stamp it and give it to a friend or relative to post back to you in a month or three months' time. It could instruct you to stick to your diet or exercise plan. It could set out health or lifestyle goals for the next month, what you expect to achieve by when. Enclose the postcard in an envelope if it's a private message. When it arrives, you'll read it, and feel the impact of the message written in your own handwriting. Choose a postcard with a picture you like, then you can stick it on the wall or a noticeboard. Every time you glance at it you'll be reminded of the message for you lurking on the other side.

■ Hang something motivational on your fridge or food cupboard. When you read it you'll think twice about opening the door and eating or drinking what's inside. That's the theory, anyway...

Read the labels of the food and drink you buy. Check out IDEA 14, *Salt away*, for a reminder about the importance of doing that.

Try another idea...

■ Create a screensaver for your PC so that every time you turn it on or leave it for a while you get a health message. This could be a holiday snap that reminds you of better times, or alternatively, the unhealthy times you're working to overcome.

■ Have a squint over the shoulder of the doctor or nurse looking at your electronic health records. They'll have highlighted the important parts of your medical history. There may be an automatic calculator on the screen capturing the health risks recorded about you. Look and learn – and pledge to minimise your health risks from then on.

■ Get a magazine about healthy living delivered regularly. Or subscribe to a journal or news sheet that maintains your interest in the healthy outdoors, helping you to plan excursions. Get hooked on a series of really useful books full of tips and ideas round health topics – so you'll look out for the next ones in the series (for example, you could check out www.52brilliantideas.com).

'*A man ought to read just as inclination leads him; for what he reads as a task will do him little good.*'
SAMUEL JOHNSON

Defining idea...

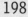

How did it go?

Q   I'm swamped by magazines, how can any one article make an impact?

A   What about arranging for a text messaging service to send you a pre-agreed reminder? How about holiday activity brochures – something you can look forward to and prepare for – as a picture and description of a mountain you'll be trekking up should get you onto the gym equipment, building up your stamina. If you love skiing, a picture of the ski slopes and the accompanying blurb should sustain your efforts to strengthen the right muscles.

Q   Is there any particular health plan I could read that you'd recommend?

A   Any plan that's been drawn up for you personally will have the most impact. Ask a personal trainer or coach at the gym to make you a plan, and take it home to re-read and think about it. You could download an individualised e-diet, tailor-made for you, from the internet.

Q   Where can I read reliable information about keeping my heart as healthy as possible?

A   There's a lot of rubbish on the internet, but lots of good stuff too. On the whole, stick with the information put out by national associations that are linked to the health and medicine professions.

45

The diary day

Accept it. You're not in control of your own life, your diary is.

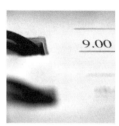

Your diary dictates when you go into work and come home, what hassles you get and how you spend your time. So make your diary work for you.

You could be jotting down what helps or stops you from taking that exercise, or eating a healthy diet. Spot a pattern and you can take action to beat it.

Make notes about what exercise you've done; what you've eaten or drunk each day. Capture how much and what kind of dedicated exercise you've taken: 'Thirty-minute power walk, forty-minute session of squash, three hour rounds of golf', etc. Tot up the calories consumed, units of alcohol drunk or any cigarettes smoked and exercise taken at the end of the week. If you're into details, compare one week with another, using bar charts or graphs. Keep your diary for several years, and you can even compare graphs from one year to another, looking for trends over time – hopefully they'll motivate you to stick with what you know is healthy for you. Here are some more ideas.

Here's an idea for you... **Spend some time tracking down contact numbers or web addresses for sources of health advice or motivation relevant to you. These could be quit smoking helplines or alcohol counselling, or maybe the numbers of friends who are trying to lose weight or get fit with you. Slip your list into the back of your diary. Then, when you're ready to seek help or tempted to revert to your bad ways, you've got instant help at hand in your diary.**

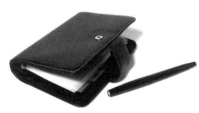

- You could choose a diary with some uplifting thoughts for the day printed at the top of each page. Read each through and reflect on what it means for you. Write your New Year resolution in your diary. Flick back to it from time to time to check if you've kept it. Make other ones, maybe on the first day of each month. Keep checking back to compare your progress on those, too.

- Now, take time to reflect on how you're doing with your healthy lifestyle. If you're cheating or breaking your pledges to yourself, think why that is happening. What is it that you can't cope with? Where are the pressures building up? That will give you new insights and help you think out solutions, which hopefully you can put in place and thereby improve your general health and your heart's chances.

- Here's a tip: a really good way to take the pressure off you is to timetable in at least 10% of your time for doing unexpected tasks. If you're in charge of how you spend your time, more or less, you'll be able to do this. That'll mean that when an emergency job crops up, or things don't go smoothly and a task takes much longer than expected, you'll be able to fit it in without stressing yourself too much. Consequently you won't have to take work home, you'll get home on time, and

Look at IDEA 41, *Break away,* **to make the most of your holiday plans.**

Try another idea...

then be able to do what you'd planned – some relaxation, exercise, sharing a meal with the family, whatever. You won't be under so much pressure, which will be good for your heart. And all thanks to your well-kept diary.

■ Having time to exercise and relax with friends doesn't 'just' happen when you're leading a frenetically busy life. You should book slots into your diary: 'Squash on Wednesdays and Sundays at 8 p.m., swimming three days a week at 7 a.m., walking the dog at 6 p.m. without fail', for example. If it's in the diary, you'll cut your other engagements to do it. If it's just a vague hope, you'll find loads of reasons to avoid doing it. Remember that old chestnut, 'Sorry, I'm too busy, I can't make it': don't let that be your slogan.

■ Holidays and weekend breaks are really important stars on the horizon of your working life to plan for and look forward to. Mark them out clearly in your diary so you preserve your time out and don't double book yourself. Highlight your holiday slots in your diary in a fluorescent marker and really savour those times ahead.

'I never travel without my diary. One should always have something sensational to read in the train.'
OSCAR WILDE

Defining idea...

How did it go?

Q   Sounds as if my diary's really crucial. What'll I do if I lose it?

A   *Consider converting your diary now from a paper version to a palmtop computer. Don't risk losing it after doing lots of work recording your exercise and diet habits, or logging your symptoms. Then you can upload what you've written to your main PC and have a regular record of your diary. And remember to back it up!*

Q   I've recently slipped up on my diet plan. We went out for a meal a month ago, then, thinking I'd broken my diet, I've been scoffing chocolates ever since. Shall I put my confessions down in my diary?

A   *Yes, it might help to log what went wrong and note your feelings. Then you can take your time pondering how to reverse your gaffe. Make a plan for recovery and enter it in your diary sheets on the relevant pages. Knowing what went wrong once should help you make sure it doesn't go wrong again.*

Q   This all sounds pretty general stuff, how can a diary help me combat the problems I have with my heart?

A   *It really helps your doctor no end if you can record information about when you have problems like chest pain or palpitations. They'll want to know how often it happened, how long it lasted, what you felt like, what helped it subside. So keep good notes in your diary and take it along to your next consultation.*

46

Early to bed

Having a heart problem does not mean the end of your sex life. Here are some tips and techniques to help you put your heart into lovemaking.

You know you're getting older when 'safe' sex means not stressing your heart so much that you get chest pain. And 'not tonight, I've got a headache' means your blood pressure's up...

Honestly, it doesn't have to be that way. Here's some help.

Yes, having sex involves physical exertion, but not much more than you need to walk up two flights of stairs. If you've got angina and can walk three hundred yards, or climb up and down two flights of stairs fairly briskly without getting any symptoms, then you should be able to have sex without bringing on your angina too, unless you're into very wild and active sex. You'll be less likely to get chest pain from your angina if you have sex at least two hours after a heavy meal or hot bath, and the room you're in is nice and warm. If having sex does trigger your angina, then relax, slow down, develop a slower and more languid style of lovemaking.

Here's an idea for you... **Do activities together with your partner that you both enjoy so you keep your relationship sparking and sexually alive. Go to the gym together, go to the cinema and sit on the back row so you can snog and hold hands, or share something exciting like your first trip in a hot air balloon.**

You might find that taking GTN beforehand, when you've not got angina, may ward off an attack and leave you to have sex in comfort.

If you seem to have lost your sex drive, or if you're a man who can't get an erection since developing angina or having a heart attack, then it may well be that you're just in the wrong frame of mind and are frightened of what may happen. There might not actually be a physical problem; anxiety and stress about the effects of your angina or heart condition can interfere in anyone's previously good sex life and suppress your and/or your partner's desire to make love. A word of warning: don't use Viagra if you take nitrate drugs for your angina – the two don't mix. Viagra can be dangerous if you've got unstable angina or had a recent heart attack, so lay off it then. Difficulties maintaining an erection can be a side effect of some drugs which are taken to lower blood pressure, or to prevent or treat angina. Go and seek help from your doctor if you've lost your libido or are having problems with impotence – the sooner the better, before it becomes a small thing (which is a big thing)

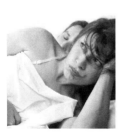

between you and your partner. Don't get depressed about it: think positively, and as you gradually gain confidence your sex life should return.

Go to **IDEA 50**, *Hearty relationships*, to think more about the benefits for your heart of having good relationships with other people as well as your partner.

Try another idea...

You might be single and looking for a new partner. Having a heart condition shouldn't stop you. Why not draw up a score card – no, not the type teenagers use to record their bonking prowess – do it like a dating agency would. Put down what you think are the essential characteristics of your potential new partner. This might be about their looks, their height or size, their food likes, how they prefer to spend their time, like how active or sporty they should be, or if they are the kind to enjoy an evening in a pub or club. Is being a non-smoker essential? Is it OK if they like a drink or two? Would you like them to be the kind to eat out or prefer a home cooked meal? Then rank your own features, and mark if they are essential or desirable for your partner. Find a new social circle or join clubs organised around some activity you like doing. Keep your score card at the front of your mind, but don't enforce every item on it – you might never be satisfied.

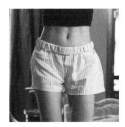 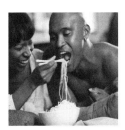

'Here's how men think. Sex, work – and those are reversible, depending on age – sex, work, food, sports and lastly, begrudgingly, relationships. And here's how women think. Relationships, relationships, relationships, work, sex, shopping, weight, food.'
CARRIE FISHER

Defining idea...

205

How did it go?

Q **Seriously, how can we relax and enjoy sex when our bones ache and we're frightened of getting angina if we over-exert ourselves?**

A *Relaxation will help. Your partner could massage your body as a preliminary to sex to help you relax. Try using some lovely oils (if they've got hard, calloused hands, the oils will make their massage smoother). Ask them to knead your back and thigh muscles. See what it takes to soothe and relax you. Return the favour and massage their body too. Work to make sex fun. Perhaps you can tell each other stories, or jokes. You could role play at being celebrities. The more fun it is, the more you'll relax and forget about any health or heart problems.*

Q **Ever since I've been on my blood pressure tablets I've difficulty getting an erection. Is it OK to leave off my tablets on the nights we have sex as my partner's getting pretty frustrated with me?**

A *It's really important to take your tablets regularly to bring your blood pressure down so that it's consistently low. It's worth swopping your tablets to find something that doesn't interfere with your erection, so talk to your doctor. You're not drowning your sorrows and drinking too much alcohol, are you? Remember that too much booze can also be a cause of impotence. Many men go on having erections into extreme old age, but those with heart disease and diabetes do have more problems.*

47

Personal aids

**There are lots of gizmos or thingummies you can use for
your personal crusade against heart disease.**

But you don't need lots. The most
effective ones are the simplest, coupled
with some good ideas to help you stay fit, slim
and healthy.

HERE ARE SOME TO HELP YOU...

- Most people who are trying to lose weight have weighing scales. These might be
  housed in the bathroom, so you can remove every gram of clothing and weigh
  yourself at your very lightest, or they might be at the gym or pharmacy. Try and
  use the type that monitors your percentage of fat and not just your total weight.
  When the scales flash up that you're made up of 40% fat or more you've got to
  accept the truth: as your new diet gets a grip, your scales will monitor your
  dwindling fat as you build up your muscles with exercise.

- Then there's your tape measure. Measure any part of your body and watch your
  shape change, especially around your waist and hips – that'll be a direct measure
  of how your risks are plummeting as you slim down.

Here's an idea for you...

If you've not got a lot of spare money, you can use an elastic band. Wind it round your packet of cigarettes, or sweets, or chocolate, or biscuits, each time you give into temptation. Then next time you crave the thing you know you should be avoiding, you have to go through the ceremony of unwinding the elastic band first. This gives you time to think, and makes it more of a conscious decision to indulge in your bad habit. Eventually you won't remove that elastic band. Then you've cracked it.

■ Now, you probably don't need a gadget to detect when you're frazzled and under stress. Just ask anybody – they can all tell you're stressed. But if you want to be a bit more scientific, wear a stress biodot inside your wrist. It changes colour according to how fast your pulse is beating as a reaction to what's going on in your life. Maybe the biodot won't change colour as you expect; you're just busy and that's why you feel under pressure, you're not over-stressed as you'd previously thought. Whatever, it'll give you more insight into how stressed you really are. Or wear a heart rate monitor on a wrist strap – and use it during your workouts too.

■ Be prepared to do exercise or play sports whenever there's an opportunity. Keep a spare sports bag and kit at the office or in the car just in case you can fit in some exercise at lunchtime. Say you finish work early, or there's a cancellation, and there's time to slip along to the club or gym or for a swim on the way home or before the next meeting – then it will be useful. Make up a compact travelling sports kit for overnight stays which you automatically take along with you, hoping you'll have time for exercising when you're away on business. Then you can just grab the kit from your car or case and you're off.

■ Keep maps available in your car that describe foot-grabbing walking routes. Then if you're away from home on business overnight, and there's time to take a walk early in the morning or evening, you know the lie of the land and where the best walks are to be had. If you're up early, maybe you'll set off walking for your first meeting, using your map, instead of taking your car to the workplace.

Getting a thorough rest has got to be good for your heart. Look at IDEA 26, *Sleep, glorious sleep*, for more on how to get a good night's sleep.

Try another idea...

■ Fix a bike rack to your car so you can stick your bicycle on, and travel out of the city to start off on a great ride in the countryside. That's much more alluring and better for you than breathing in car fumes on congested roads, which are bad for your heart. Or buy a folding bike. Then take that with you to the big city so you can cycle onwards from the train, or park your car and ride to your final destination on your bike. Wear a face mask to partly protect you from the fumes. Your folding bike should pay for itself in no time, saving you petrol costs, horrendous car parking charges, taxi bills or public transport tickets.

■ Position a piece of simple exercise equipment in every room of your home. Then you can pop on your bike or rowing machine or whatever for a few minutes here and there. It all adds up.

'Help yourself, and heaven will help you.'
JEAN DE LA FONTAINE, French writer

Defining idea...

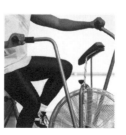

How did it go?

Q How can I resist the temptations at birthdays and Christmas when everyone gives me chocolates and wine as presents – and I feel obliged to eat and drink them?

A   *What about writing out a list like engaged couples do, to suggest wedding presents they'd like? Your nearest and dearest will be glad to know what it is you want. Give them a specific list of the health books you want, the calorie reference book, the running shoes or sports equipment, or a bad weather kit so you can still keep fit when it's wet. What about stocking up on a steamer or a lean grilling machine?*

Q That's fine, but it's not just the stuff I get. You know what it's like – there are always things about that I shouldn't be touching. Is there anything else can I do?

A   *Well, you don't need an expensive gadget to help your willpower. Use mementos or trophies as personal aids to reinforce good ways to behave and minimise risks for your heart. These could be pictures of a slim and fit you stuck up somewhere where you'll see them every day, or certificates of achievement – maybe for winning a sports competition, even for something like ballroom dancing. Take a good look at them and they should strengthen your resolve.*

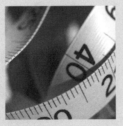 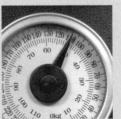

48

About time

Some time pressure is necessary to maintain your interest in getting a job done, but you need to learn how to relax as well.

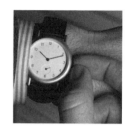

Too much pressure can tip you over your peak so that you're less efficient, less effective all round and your heart suffers. So balance your work and leisure time.

Anyone can get in a mess with their schedule. Here are some basic ideas to help you get yours right, and minimise the stress to your heart as well.

- Give yourself enough free time every day for rest and relaxation outside your working hours, to counteract the stresses and strains of your working life. Don't take work home. Otherwise you'll become stale and miserable.

- Keeping a daily log of how you spend your time for a week or so will check that you're protecting enough time for yourself. Can you honestly say you've spent a few hours this week doing something just for *your own* enjoyment or leisure?

Here's an idea for you...

Try and delegate as much of your work as you can to someone else – why do it if you don't have to? If you're the poor person that other people delegate work to, make sure you understand what's required, and that you've the time, skills and experience to do it. You'll just waste time if you don't know what you're supposed to be doing or how to set about doing it. If you don't have the skills for it, insist on getting the training you'll need first. And don't forget to ask for a pay rise at the same time!

■ Prioritise how you spend your time. Don't allow yourself (or other people) to waste it. Have you got clear goals for your work or career or your home life, or for your leisure or sport? How you allot your time will look very different if you intend being a great golfer, or learning a new skill such as aromatherapy or getting an educational qualification, or spending as much time as possible with your family. You'll want to discuss and refine your goals with whoever else they affect. Then make sure that your various goals don't conflict, or else you'll never get there. When there's a choice about how you spend your time, match the possible activities against your goals; if they take you further away from them, then refuse to do those activities; but if they bring you closer to achieving your goals, see if you've got time to fit them in. Get into the habit of regarding minutes or hours as costed time; this lets you rate how much the different activities on which you spend time are worth, and whether they are all of equal value.

Defining idea...

'Procrastination is the thief of time.'
Proverb

■ Distasteful or complicated tasks are the ones you'll be more likely to put off. But if it's essential or important, you'll have to do it sometime, and you'll only feel guilty postponing it. If you wait too long the job will be even more difficult, as you'll forget your previous ideas or what the instructions were. Wait until you've time to complete the job before you start on it.

You can 'stress-proof' yourself. Look at IDEA 25, *Break with stress*, to learn more stress-busting techniques.

Try another idea...

Don't pick up a piece of paper and half read it, decide it's too difficult to tackle or you haven't enough time and put it aside. You'll have wasted the time you spent deciding to put it off. Try and get yourself geared up for the job, launch into it and then complete it. Train yourself to do the tedious or horrible task first, then reward yourself straight afterwards with another job you really want to do – or by having some fun time, not chocolate!

- If you're an extrovert you'll be revitalised from brainstorming and discussions with others, and that will be the most efficient way to spend your time. If you're more of an introvert you'll want time to sit and think and read. Whichever is your way, make sure you get enough of it to replenish your creativity and enthusiasm.

- One of the secrets of a happy life is to get the balance of stress right. You want just enough stress to give you a zing, but not so much as to make work and life seem an endless grind that burns you out and strains your heart. So make regular time for fun, relaxation, hobbies and enjoying simple pleasures.

After all, you need to be fresh and creative to stay on top of the demands made on you at work and home, for your heart's sake. If you keep on overworking, it will just be counterproductive in the end.

'Men talk of killing time, while time quietly kills them.' DION BOUCICAULT, nineteenth-century playwright

Defining idea...

How did
it go?

**Q   It's all very well to say I've got to prioritise what I do but what can
you do when everyone wants a piece of you, and pushes jobs and
demands on you?**

A   *You've just got to learn to be assertive, to say no often enough to
unnecessary work, taking on other people's jobs or the family's tasks or
duties. Think of their side of it – if you're mug enough to do things for
them, then that saves them asking or paying someone else to do it. They'll
just carry on dumping jobs on you, and making you feel guilty if you don't
get on with them.*

**Q   My partner wastes lots of time going over the past and wondering
if he's made the right decisions. That's no way to be going on, is
it? How can he move forward?**

A   *Here's some general advice that might help him, and you, come to that.
When you have to make a decision, gather information about the problem
or choice, weigh up the pros and cons and make the decision. That's it.
Once you've made that decision, look forward and make plans for the
future; don't look backwards and go on and on about your regrets. Put any
past mistakes behind you and don't ruminate over them.*

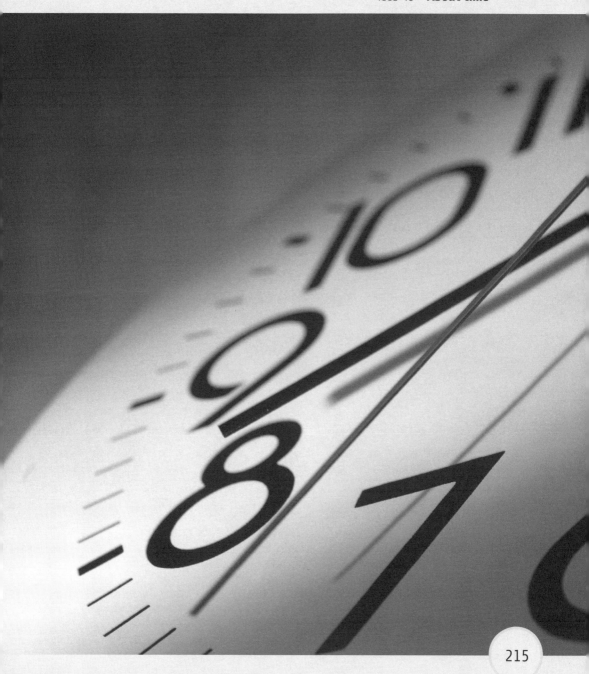

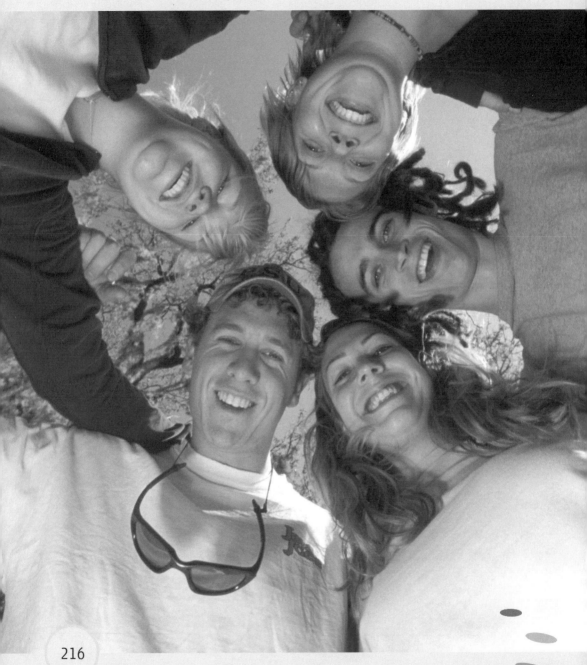

49

You're in good company

Being a groupie is not just about hanging around after celebrities; belonging to a group might help your own feel-good factor.

Losing weight, stopping smoking, resisting alcohol, getting fit — all are much easier to do with other people than when you're struggling on your own.

Get hold of a few friends and make up your own group, or find one you can join. Then there'll be others to keep you on the straight and narrow, whatever you decide to do, who you'll have to face up to if you start cheating on your healthy resolve. They can give you a bit of competition, maybe to see who can lose the most weight or run the furthest or fastest – and can also keep up your interest in what you're doing. You can all make a pact and agree your joint goals. Maybe you could publicise your goals if you are earning money for charity as a result. You won't be able to let the others down, then. And give the members of your group official permission to embarrass you if you slip up, by a notice on the office wall, for example. You can also plan to celebrate your success together – putting up a banner or a holding a party when you reach your goals.

Here's an idea for you...

Book a club holiday where you'll have guaranteed company on any number of outdoor activities. Go on your own, or maybe with your partner, friends or family joining in with the group on all sorts of new and energetic activities. A word of warning: don't be seduced by the group into undoing the good work on your fitness with drinking or eating too much when you're relaxing in the evening. Trying out a new sport or activity could give you a taste for it, so that you seek out a local club when you're back home again, keeping up the activity and maintaining your fitness with the support and camaraderie of new friends.

Defining idea...

'Take the tone of the company you are in.'
LORD CHESTERFIELD, eighteenth-century writer

You can get some of the same effects with just one other person. Keep up with a particular buddy who's getting healthy with you, or someone who's interested in your well-being. Telephone, text and email each other to chat through temptations and progress, and draw on each other's experience. Don't be shy about asking for their help. You can motivate each other and keep reinforcing what you've got to gain by tackling your (mutual) weaknesses. Go and see them for a chat to stop yourself raiding the fridge or popping out to buy bottles of drink or boxes of chocolate.

Home alone? You know that alone you're inclined to be weak; there's no one to see you have that quick smoke, criticise you for eating those snacks or downing that beer. So don't spend too much time on your own. If you know that you usually break your resolve when you stay at home on your own all evening, then invite friends round, arrange to go out with others to see a film – get others on your side, watching and briefing you. Arrange to do something active regularly with someone else if you can – like walking your dogs together, or taking a power walk round the streets to get you out and about. And don't forget that there are loads of telephone or internet helplines to support you if you're trying to stop smoking or lose weight, beat depression, etc. Seek out ones to suit you and your health or lifestyle challenge and see if they have call-back facilities, or offer motivational counsellors, or can just give you the information you want.

You could even find a benefactor who'll bribe you to be good! A parent, maybe, even your partner? Agree what it is you're to achieve – and what the reward will be. Maybe you have several milestones and an overall goal that'll be difficult to reach but not impossible. Keep visualising the rewards and what you stand to lose if you don't make your goal. If you're a selfless person, motivated by helping others, then there's no reason why your reward can't be something to benefit other people rather than yourself.

You'll never walk alone if you join a rambling association or walking club; see IDEA 5, *Step outside*, for more on the benefits of walking, and IDEA 27, *Health at work*, for advice on group activities there.

Try another idea...

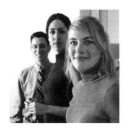

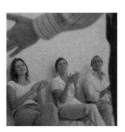

'Please accept my resignation. I don't want to belong to any club that will accept me as a member.'
GROUCHO MARX

Defining idea...

How did it go?

Q   **Is it better to stick with a group than try and do it on my own in order to beat my weight problem?**

A   *If you're a pretty private person, you'll probably find it difficult to bare your soul and innermost thoughts about your eating habits to relative strangers. But, on the whole, if you've relapsed in the past or find it difficult to keep your promises to yourself to eat a balanced diet or lead a more healthy life, then it's time to try involving other people. They'll support you – and you them – through a slimming club: or use the internet as an alternative.*

Q   **I get angina, so do you think if I joined a fitness group at my health club I'd end up pushing myself too far, beyond what's good for me?**

A   *Exercise isn't ruled out; in fact it's the norm to do cardiac rehabilitation even after a heart attack in a special gym, where the same people see each other week after week even if they're not doing group activities. So find some other friends with similar health problems and make sure you all visit the gym at certain times so you've got each other's friendship and support. But you're right to be wary of pushing yourself beyond your capacity. Get some professional advice from the fitness trainers at your gym.*

50

Hearty relationships

You're not sailing solo round the world, so you've no choice but to get on with others. Your relationships with them will keep you in good heart – and might even save your life.

Everyone knows that love makes you feel better and live longer. Love and friendship are good for your heart, to keep it in tip-top condition whatever your age or state of health.

Everyone needs personal networks. Have you people in your life with whom you give and receive affection and love? If so, make the most of those relationships. If not, get out there and make new friends or find a new partner. You need a dynamic network of supportive friends and colleagues because times change, people move on, and you mature and develop. Maintain and renew your networks or they'll go stale, and you will be out of touch or bored with them.

Try and inject some freshness into your relationship with your partner. Make a date, as in the old days, and try to arrange regular outings doing shared activities or interests. See if you can revitalise your sex life, if it's suffered because you're not communicating and spending too little time alone together. Make your relationship

Here's an idea for you...

Set yourself a month's trial for saying how you feel. Sharing thoughts and feelings is a must for any meaningful relationship. Try at least three different situations where you're in a one-to-one position with someone else – with the family at home, with a friend or a colleague at work. Try saying 'You make me feel...' and then make a factual statement. Keep it positive; don't be judgemental, as that will just put the other person's hackles up. And if you adopt a professional mask at work you can forget to remove it when you go home. Hiding your expression and feelings can mean you're perceived as a cold fish, not compassionate or caring as, of course, you really are.

with your partner a priority and you'll have lots of fun and love which will keep your heart healthy.

Make time so that your children have your full attention. Show genuine interest in what they've been up to and praise them when you can. Talk about your work with them so they can be more understanding about your being away from home, if that's a feature of your working life. Re-evaluate the commitments that are keeping you away from your family, especially if these are in the evenings, at nights or at weekends, and see if you can drop or change any. Find ways of having fun as a family and growing together that will stay with you the rest of your lives.

Do be careful at work, because the closer your relationships are with your customers or clients, the more it drains you – so try and limit their intensity. Obviously, if you never interact and 'give yourself' in any way, your work would be dissatisfying and that could be a source of stress in itself. But the inverse is also true, so guard against becoming too involved with your clients' problems and emotions. Otherwise, you may find that your own family life suffers as you become emotionally drained with too little energy left for exchanging love and support with your loved ones.

If your job's not the right one for you, then check out IDEA 28, *Work at it*, and have a rethink.

Try another idea...

Being self-aware will help you. Some people are unaware of their own emotions, motivations and attitudes. You'll be familiar with some of your behaviours, feelings and thoughts, as will your partner and other people. You'll have some blind spots, and there'll be some emotions and behaviour you choose to keep hidden. If you want to develop more self-awareness begin with listening to yourself, your thoughts, feelings and your reasons for particular behaviour. Listen and learn from what other people, like your family or colleagues, can tell you about yourself. Don't bottle your emotions up but reveal your feelings and thoughts to others in your immediate circle. Denial is a powerful defence mechanism you might be using unconsciously – denial of the dangers of smoking or overeating, for instance. You may pretend to yourself that all is well. People who are dependent on drugs or alcohol often have little insight into their addiction. They feel they're in control of their drinking and deny it affects their work... and this is where self-awareness kicks in.

'Women deprived of the company of men pine, men deprived of the company of women become stupid.'
ANTON CHEKHOV

Defining idea...

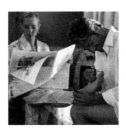

How did
it go?

Q **I find it difficult to express my feelings – what hope is there for me?**

A *Maybe expressing your feelings in non-verbal ways would be easier than being direct about how you're feeling. Do that through the colour of your clothes – brighten them up, perhaps – or use a creative hobby as a medium. It might be the way you carry yourself, or sit or stand, and the type of body language you use that conveys your meaning.*

Q **I'm starting a new job tomorrow as a manager in a new company, my first promotion and it's a bit scary. How can I create the right environment for the staff to work together, as the customers can be stroppy?**

A *Cultivate a really supportive culture. But too much social grazing can interfere with output at work and distract people from their jobs, so help your staff get the right balance between friendliness (or gossip) and getting on with their work. Perhaps you can set up a system of debriefing if a customer gets you all worked up – to help shed and share the stress and worry, and move on.*

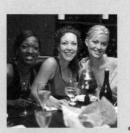

51

Relaxing you

Relaxation is good for your heart. It's a skill that you can learn in order to slow your heart rate and lower your blood pressure.

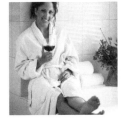

Do remember, everything in moderation — you wouldn't want to be so relaxed all the time that you achieved nothing. Here are some ideas for 'alternative' ways to relax.

- Learning to relax while visualising events you fear can help you to control the feelings provoked in the real situation that triggers stress or anxiety for you. Try different forms of relaxation like meditation, yoga or self-hypnosis to find the method that suits you.

- Positive visualisation can help you to relax and feel happy. A picture of a favourite pet strategically placed in your office can distract you from the day's woes. Keep small items nearby that have a special meaning for you, such as a ticket to a play, a champagne cork, or something the kids made for you, so as to be able to recall a cherished memory and – relax.

Here's an idea for you...

Listening to relaxation tapes or CDs can have a soothing and calming influence on one person, and be intensely irritating to another. It depends on your personal preferences and styles. Why not buy a relaxation tape and see if it's helpful for you? Please don't listen to the tape while driving the car, though, in case it makes you sleepy and less alert than usual. Choose a time and place when you're unlikely to be disturbed, lie back in an armchair or stretch out on a comfortable settee or bed, and play the tape through twice. This may seem an easy way to manage stress, but it's not. If you're someone who finds it difficult to relax, who becomes fidgety if they're waiting around with nothing to do, you'll have to be very firm with yourself to listen quietly to the whole tape.

■ Acupuncture is another way to tackle stress and anxiety. In general, acupuncture has a sedating effect. Acupuncture points run along 'meridian' channels. Needles are inserted into specific designated points on the body relating to any particular problems you're experiencing. Stimulation from the needle points redirects channels of energy beneath the skin to restore your body's energy levels (called *qi* or *chi*) and create 'harmony' in your normal bodily functions. There are specific points on the top of your head and on your ear that the acupuncturist can use to induce relaxation.

■ You'll feel very relaxed after a reflexology session. Reflexology is a form of therapeutic massage to areas of your feet in order to produce specific beneficial effects in other parts of your body. The underside of your foot is like a chart of your whole body, and there are specific reflex points on your feet which correspond to certain parts of it: bones, muscles, organs, glands, circulation and nerve pathways. The practitioner's thumb and finger pressure on your feet will release any tension and unblock previously 'stuck' energy. They'll massage both your feet in this way to treat your body as a whole.

- Aromatherapy is good for relieving anxiety, nausea and stress-related conditions, as well as giving pain relief. It's generally given as a course of treatment so that the benefits can take root. As time goes by, you'll feel more relaxed. The benefits of aromatherapy come from the natural healing properties of the oils that are used. These oils may be extracted from flowers, leaves, fruit, stems, wood, bark, resin or roots. Essential oils are around seventy times more concentrated than raw parts of the parent plants, and aromatherapy oils are usually massaged in. But they can also be added as a few drops to your bath, or used as a perfume, an inhalant, a compress, a vaporiser or room spray.

Holidays are good for relaxing, but they're also an ideal opportunity to try out new ways of doing that. Check out IDEA 41, Break away.

Try another idea...

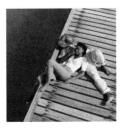

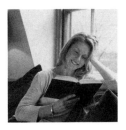

'Natural forces within us are the true healers of disease.'
HIPPOCRATES

Defining idea...

Q **I'm so busy with my family and job and keeping up the garden and house that I've just too little time to relax, though I'd love to. What's the quickest way?**

A *Remember you? The person with whom you live twenty-four hours a day? Sounds like you need to prioritise some time for yourself, and not put everyone else first all the time. Book yourself a day out at a health club and try some of their relaxing treatments (then work out a plan for more, much, much more, while you're under their influence!). Make the most of any slack time to relax. Even if it's while you're trapped at rail crossings, in traffic jams or supermarket queues or even washing up: get into the habit of switching off completely from your worries and hassles, and thinking relaxing private thoughts.*

Q **What's a healthy way of relaxing after a hard day's work?**

A *If you're a competitive type of person, then relaxation could mean doing your usual sport or pastime at sub-maximal speed: a ramble rather than a sprint, or a slow crawl rather than swimming against the clock. Or you might interpret 'complete relaxation' as being transposed to an entirely passive state, away from pressure and hassles, listening to music or a relaxation tape. A glass or two of alcohol might help – keeping within your day's healthy allowance and, of course, if you're not driving later. You could keep one room in your house for relaxing purposes. Bar any work being taken in there by anyone. Then, when you go and sit in that room you'll automatically relax, associating the place with pleasant, relaxing feelings.*

You know it...

You're not going to become a saint overnight. But there's so much you can do to improve the health of your heart.

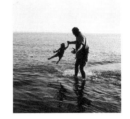

Don't despair if you relapse and undo some of the good changes you've made to your lifestyle... At least your health benefited yesterday.

Think things through, and fire up your good intentions again.

The very first part of making a change is understanding why you should. Maybe you see no problem, but other people tell you there's an issue – perhaps you're smoking or drinking too much alcohol or ignoring the health dangers of being overweight. Understanding is the first part, but believing you can change is the second stage. This is when you weigh up the pros and cons of taking action. Next, be more aware of what you are doing – your own behaviours – so you can plan what to do about it. Then, become more aware of what you are thinking. Try and block 'bad' thoughts, and put your positive thoughts and determination into perspective. Start planning changes you're going to make, and remember: understanding, believing, doing and thinking are key.

Here's an idea for you...

Capture those moments when you suddenly see the light, when health messages really do get through to you and penetrate your shell. Maybe your dentist tells you about the damage all those toffees are doing to your teeth, maybe you run for the train or bus and miss it because you're not as fit as you used to be. Or perhaps a close relative dies from heart disease and you realise you might be next. Write down how you feel. Record your thoughts, talking through your good intentions and promises, and then your action plan for changing things. Keep replaying that recording until you have actually made those changes to reinforce your new ways.

Your personality is what differentiates you from someone else. It's made up from the three components of thinking or beliefs, feelings, and attitudes. People with strongly competitive personalities demand a lot of themselves and others. They drive themselves on, and expect perfection – at home, at work and in personal relationships. If you're like this, be aware that these characteristics may be harmful, even altering the cholesterol level in your blood and making you more prone to having a heart attack. It is possible to modify your competitive behaviour. And if you tend to be self-critical too, then you'll be even more prone to stress and depression.

Now, compulsivity is a common personality trait, particularly associated with doubt, guilt feelings and an exaggerated sense of responsibility. If you're a workaholic, and you've got a compulsive nature, then you'll typically react by working even harder rather than taking time off to relax. Again, think seriously about trying to moderate this tendency.

Don't forget that it's impossible to be a perfect parent, perfect wife or husband, perfect teacher or manager or whatever you are at work. Something has to go. If you're a perfectionist you'll be unhappy that you can't be perfect in all your roles and responsibilities – it's just not possible. Next thing you know you'll be eating or smoking for comfort, or brewing up a heart attack because of all the tensions and guilt you're feeling. Forgive yourself for not being perfect and think whether the failings you criticise or mock in others are what you dislike about yourself. You can change, and you know it... give it a try.

Check out IDEA 3, *New You resolution*, and decide to be more active or change another aspect of your lifestyle. You can do it, you know you can.

Try another idea...

This should help. Build your confidence and self-esteem. If you need permission to look after yourself and admit that you have needs, here it is: your official permission. Now write your worries down on a piece of paper and then symbolically throw them away. Prepare well for any situations you're going to find yourself in – new relationships, interviews, a new job, being a parent or grandparent for the first time, and give yourself every opportunity to succeed. If you know your own personality and needs then organise things so you feel comfortable whenever possible – for example, if you're an introvert don't force yourself unnecessarily into situations that only an extrovert would enjoy.

In brief, learn from any mistakes or failures so that you know how to succeed next time. And don't set yourself up to fail; you don't have to!

'Only the most intelligent and the most stupid do not change.'
CONFUCIUS

Defining idea...

231

How did it go?

Q **I'm a hopeless case, full of good intentions but they always fizzle out. I end up even fatter and smoking more and more. What can I do?**

A *Learn to ignore each relapse. OK, you've worked out your good intentions – now tell everybody. Let your friends and family watch you and help keep you on the straight and narrow. If you slip up once, that's no big deal. You haven't undone all your last few weeks good behaviour with that one slip, so forgive yourself. I know that's easier said than done, but you can do it, if you want to enough.*

Q **I've read lots about staying healthy. Where do I start when there's so much information out there?**

A *Don't let the plethora of health information be an excuse to stop you from getting on with converting to a healthy lifestyle. You shouldn't use information overload as an excuse to let you off trying to stay healthy and improve your lifestyle. When you're in your nineties and still healthy, you'll look happily back at how you put wise health advice into practice and bore everyone by retelling your 'be like me' stories.*

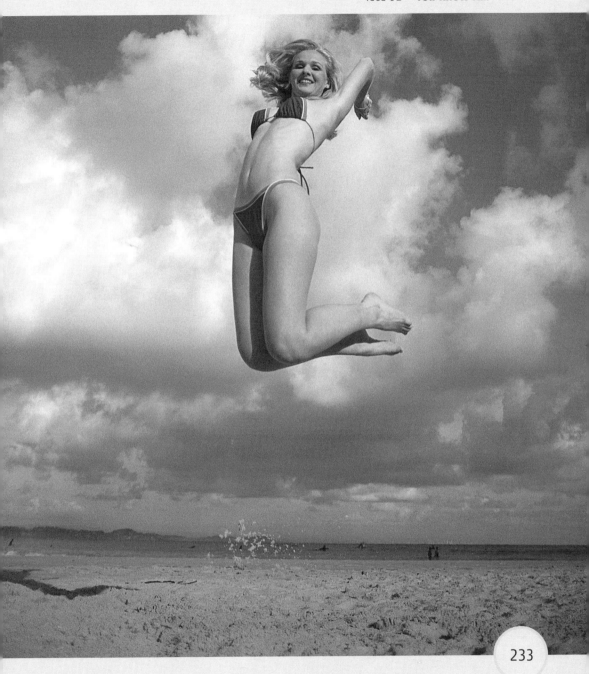

The end...

Or is it a new beginning? We hope that the ideas in this book will have inspired you to try some new things to heal your aching heart. We hope you've found that making small but effective lifestyle changes has worked and that you're already stubbing out the cigarettes, walking the dog every day and stocking your fridge with hearty, nutritious food. You should be well on your way to a healthier, fitter, more fulfilled and balanced you, brimming with good intentions.

You're mean, you're motivated and you don't care who knows it.

So why not let us know all about it? Tell us how you got on. What did it for you – what really got the blood pumping through your veins? Maybe you've got some tips of your own you want to share (see next page if so). And if you liked this book you may find we have even more brilliant ideas that could change other areas of your life for the better.

You'll find the Infinite Ideas crew waiting for you online at www.infideas.com.

Or if you prefer to write, then send your letters to:
Healthy Heart
The Infinite Ideas Company Ltd
36 St Giles, Oxford OX1 3LD, United Kingdom

We want to know what you think, because we're all working on making our lives better too. Give us your feedback and you could win a copy of another *52 Brilliant Ideas* book of your choice. Or maybe get a crack at writing your own.

Good luck. Be brilliant.

Offer one

CASH IN YOUR IDEAS

We hope you enjoy this book. We hope it inspires, amuses, educates and entertains you. But we don't assume that you're a novice, or that this is the first book that you've bought on the subject. You've got ideas of your own. Maybe our author has missed an idea that you use successfully. If so, why not send it to yourauthormissedatrick@infideas.com, and if we like it we'll post it on our bulletin board. Better still, if your idea makes it into print we'll send you four books of your choice or the cash equivalent. You'll be fully credited so that everyone knows you've had another Brilliant Idea.

Offer two

HOW COULD YOU REFUSE?

Amazing discounts on bulk quantities of Infinite Ideas books are available to corporations, professional associations and other organisations.

For details call us on:
+44 (0)1865 514888
Fax: +44 (0)1865 514777
or e-mail: info@infideas.com

Where it's at...